CW01559035

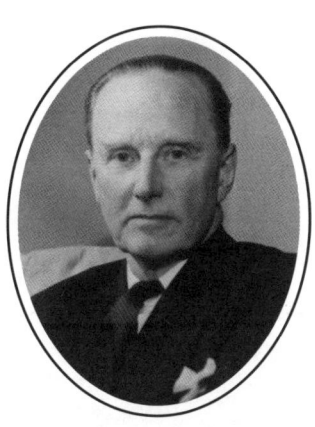

Wilfred Fish
and a profession in the making

J D Manson

19 | 5 | 03.
From the Publisher
Invoice 17.
£22-35

Publisher
Esmeralda Press
12 Wheatley Street
London W1G 8PS

Design and production
Western Arts
020 8341 1248

© J D Manson 2003

ISBN 0-9536102-1-7

To my wife

CONTENTS

PREFACE

Early in 1959 I travelled from Leeds, where I had been in general dental practice for over ten years, to London, and from Kings Cross to Lincoln's Inn Fields to see Sir Wilfred Fish at the Royal College of Surgeons. The last time I had visited those dignified portals was to collect my Fellowship, and thereby to reinforce my aspiration to specialise in periodontology. In Britain at that time there was no formal pathway to specialisation except in oral surgery and orthodontics, and knowing no-one who could advise me I wrote to Sir Wilfred, who agreed immediately to see me.

My training at Leeds Dental School in my chosen speciality was negligible. As students we were taught that gingivitis and pyorrhoea were caused by calculus, seen in gross abundance in our patients. There was little or no teaching of the pathology of these diseases, indeed they were a mystery, and treatment centred on scaling and extraction. Gross oral sepsis was common and dental diseases, both caries and periodontal disease, were rampant. The 'gas room' was the busiest place in the school, and we students competed for first place in the race to extract a thousand teeth.

Then in 1944 the first edition of 'Parodontal Disease; A Manual of Treatment and Atlas of Pathology' by E. Wilfred Fish appeared. If my memory serves me correctly it was introduced to our teachers by Bryan Wade, then a senior student who was to become my boss at the Royal Dental Hospital. He had the advantage that his father was a dentist. In practice the book became my bible. I followed Fish's treatment plans step by step; I bought Fish gingivectomy knives, and my nurse became an expert in mixing his recommended surgical dressing of Zinc Oxide, Oil of Cloves and shredded cotton wool. My patients became propagandists for gingival massage with balsa wood dental sticks. I was saving teeth, at least for a while and then not always. A decade in practice is long enough to test one's ability to obtain success with any technique, and despite my and the patient's best efforts I failed too frequently for my satisfaction. It seemed to me that more had to be learned.

Sir Wilfred received me with courtesy and without any condescension, and immediately introduced me to Bert Cohen, and to the focus of their current research on the aetiology of periodontal disease, the interdental col, about which they both waxed lyrical. In short I was treated as a professional equal.

The past fifty years have witnessed a transformation in the dental scene of this country. The prevalence of both dental caries and periodontal diseases has dropped dramatically, gross oral sepsis is rare, dental health is valued and the words, oral hygiene and bacterial plaque, are familiar to the public at large. Concurrently the independence of the dental profession has been largely established, and in all these changes Fish played a major role; as a scientist, an administrator, a political activist for his profession, a hospital consultant and a general dental practitioner of extraordinary ability as examples of his work at the Odontological Museum show. He bestrode the dental arena, and it is in recognition of that fact that I have attempted to tell Fish's story, which, to use his words, is also that of a profession in the making.

In this venture I have had enormous help and encouragement from many people, in particular from Lady Hazel Fish and Professor Bert Cohen, who knew Fish the man as well as the professional person better than anyone. In that context I would like to thank Professor A.E.W. (Loma) Miles, who provided me with those insights that only a perceptive student has of his teacher. Graeme Stewart Ross , who as a boy knew Fish well and Mrs. Molly Goulding, Fish's secretary for some years, were also very helpful in giving me their personal views of the man.

Bert Cohen, Stephen Hancocks and Stuart McKenzie (who also provided much information about Fish at Manchester and at the British Society of Periodontology), have been strict and therefore immensely valuable editors of the whole manuscript, and I have profited from useful criticism readily provided by Professor Barry Eley, Sir Ian Gainsford, Professor Stanley Gelbier, Mr. George Kantorowicz, Sir David Mason, Professor David Poswillo.

Fish's grandson, Judge Rodney Greaves, and grand-daughter,

Trich Bezuidenhout have supplied me with essential information about the family, and I am indebted to Mr. Lawrence Baker of Perth, West Australia, for putting me in touch with this now far-flung generation; to Louis Nagy and Stuart Oakenfull who have been unstinting in their co-operation in opening the files of the Sevenoaks practice founded by Fish, and now flourishing as Eustace and Partners, and to Tony Fish (no relative) of the Chevening Estate Office in Sevenoaks, who found data on Fish's early homes in that town.

In writing about the Royal Dental Hospital I have relied heavily on the London Metropolitan Archives and on 'The History of the Royal Dental Hospital of London and School of Dental Surgery 1858-1985' by Ernest G. Smith and Beryl D. Cottell, to whom I owe many thanks. I am grateful to Ben Fickling and Douglas Munns for accounts of the early department of Periodontology at the R.D.H., and to Professor John Eastoe, Dr.William Bowen and Professor Newell Johnson, who added invaluable information to that of Professor Cohen's, about the research at the Department of Dental Science.

My progress in researching information would have been much more difficult without the willing help of Mr. Roger Farby and his staff at the BDA Information Centre, of Mrs. Muriel Cohen, widow of the respected dental historian, Ronald Cohen, and that of Roxane Fea, Head of the BDA Museum Service, and I am grateful to Mike Grace, editor of the British Dental Journal, for permission to quote many passages from that journal.

I would like to thank Mrs. Tina Craig, Librarian at the Royal College of Surgeons, for her almost daily help with the Fish archive and the RCS for kind permission to use photographs from the archives, as well as Simon Chaplin, Senior Curator of RCS Museums; also Kevin Brown, the archivist at St. Mary's Hospital, David Martin Brown of Kingswood School, for their unfailing assistance, Allen Packwood at the Churchill Archive and Sir Martin Gilbert for information about Churchill's dental treatment. The Wellcome Library provided me with access to the fascinating Mellanby archive with its detailed documentation of research in-fighting. Reverend J. Martin Bailey and Dr. Dorothy Graham, helped me understand something of the Wesleyan faith; Kate S. Wood, at the archives of the Imperial War Museum assisted me to unearth data on Captain E.W. Fish; and the staff of the General Dental Council helped with the activity of the Dental Board. Sarah Wartes of the Bayler College of Dentistry and George Kantorowicz provided me with information about Dr. Bernhard Gottlieb of Vienna, from whom Fish learned so much.

Finally I would like to acknowledge my debt to the late Professor H.M. Pickard. 'Pick' had plans to write the biography of his teacher, friend and inspiration, and I feel sure that if fate had allowed he would have written an elegant account; as it was the notes that he gave me provided me with a valuable start to this tribute to a man whom I consider to be, with Sir John Tomes the stars of my profession.

J.D.M.

INTRODUCTION

"A hundred years in the affairs of a nation or of a profession is a canvas wide enough to permit the trend of evolution to be depicted. On it may be recorded the outline of significant successes or of no less importance failures in their approximate perspective. This is particularly so in our own profession for the foundations of its modern structure were only just being laid a century ago."

So began a talk entitled, "The Englishman's teeth" read by Dr. E.Wilfred Fish, M.D., D.D.S., D.Sc. to the West Lancashire and West Cheshire Branch of the British Dental Association on November 22, 1941.

In this solemn, almost Churchillian, introduction, Fish was certainly mindful of the affairs of the nation at that time; the beginning of the third year of the second Great War in a generation. Hitler dominated Europe and four-months earlier had invaded the Soviet Union. The German armies had moved so quickly that by November they were on the outskirts of Moscow. A puppet French government was installed at Vichy, and De Gaulle with the Free French army had escaped to England. More immediately ominous, German submarines were enjoying huge success in the Atlantic destroying Britain's merchant fleet and endangering the supply of food and essential raw materials.

Only a few weeks earlier (October 29) in a talk at his alma mater, Harrow School, the Prime Minister, Winston Churchill, Fish's patient for many years, had said," Do not let us speak of darker days; let us rather speak of sterner days." Many of the younger generation of dentists were in the armed forces, as Fish like many in the hall, had been in the First War, and his audience, aware of Churchill's words, will have been a mature and sombre group. Fish was then in the Home Guard as a Captain and medical advisor to the Kent zone.

Fish had certainly chosen the title and theme of his talk to reflect the mood of national solidarity. The profession was still fragmented by virtue of qualification and experience, even by social status, but at the meeting '1921 men' rubbed shoulders with fellow professionals with letters after their names, and 'honoraries', the senior members of the profession who operated at local hospitals.

Fish's national and international reputation as a scientist and clinician was well established, and two years earlier he had been elected to the Dental Board of the United Kingdom, the predecessor of the present General Dental Council. He could command the respect and attention of his audience whatever their status in the profession. His talk encompassed the scientific and clinical evolution of the dental profession against the social and medical background of its time, and in its breadth of vision and elegant presentation it was a portent of his rise to the top of the profession. In playing a major role in translating dentistry from a craft to a profession, Fish is regarded by many as one of the most influential figure in British dentistry in the twentieth century.

Over one hundred years earlier a cartoon drawn by George Cruikshank shows vividly the contemporary image of the dentist. Standing on a stool with his powerful back towards us, he is spread across a struggling lady patient who in her agony has kicked over the dentist's trolley, under which a startled little dog is barking. Instruments are sent flying and in the doorway there is a figure of an onlooker, aghast and frightened. It is a picture of pain and terror and an event to be avoided at all costs.

Such pictures, memorably drawn by famous political cartoonists such as Gilray and Rowlandson, were immensely popular in the eighteenth and nineteenth centuries all over Europe. Many showed the tooth-puller operating in fairgrounds or blacksmith's forges. Indeed anyone who considered himself capable of pulling teeth usually as a sideline occupation, whether he be surgeon, apothecary, barber or blacksmith was free to do so.

A signboard of the time from Ottery St. Mary, Devon reads:

> "The Smith-Glazier; Let Blood and Draws
> Teeth, Tea Kittels & Potts, Buckets, Lantern
> Cups to be Handled Here."

An article in the New York Mirror (14 March, 1835) stated, "Any person who can possess him of a key and a few scrapers is at liberty to do what seems good to him to the ivories of all who have courage enough to instruct themselves in his hands."

The reputation of the dentist was as a charlatan and even crook.

In an early Dutch etching by Lucas van Leyden (1523) entitled The Charlatan, the tooth-puller is at work while his assistant rifles the victim's pockets.

Early in the nineteenth century, it was seen to be essential for respectable practitioners in the USA and Europe to free their profession from the stigma of association with the multitude of such charlatans. Although the motivation and aspirations of dentists in the USA and in Britain were the same, the pioneers in these countries trod quite different paths. As Fish said in the 1941 lecture, change came, "slowly and painfully in this country, but more obviously and speedily in America....".

Britain lagged behind the Continent and the USA in formalising its medical and dental professions. While in France L'Ecole Dentaire had been founded in 1699, and the legalising of the dental surgeon followed soon after, Britain had to wait almost two hundred years to gain a legitimately recognised dental profession.

In the USA, the practical and mechanical aspects of professional activity were highly valued. In the climate of the time before the American Civil War, concern with practical results dominated thinking. The telegraph, the railroad, sewing machine, combined harvester, were manifestations of innovation to achieve practical results.

Such thinking also underlay changes in medical practise, but as a largely technical discipline, dentistry was especially open to technical innovation. The denture that could stay in place without springs, improved ivory teeth, the dental use of vulcanised rubber, better designed forceps and cavity preparation that would retain fillings, often of gold foil, as well as variously constructed crowns, all these and many more technical advances brought benefits to the dental patient.

In the USA sentiment among dentists ran against a close association of medical and dental education. Although many favoured a general medical education, many dentists did not feel that physicians had sufficient appreciation of the "dental art" and the need for emphasis on technique and innovation in restorative dentistry and prosthetics as well as orthodontics. Today, dentistry in the USA is an autonomous profession separate from that of medicine, and dental schools are always autonomous from medical schools. There is no medical school with a dental department, and even in the nineteenth century where such an arrangement obtained it eventually collapsed.

In the field of public health, dentistry is administered separately from that of medicine, and in the US Public Health Service there is a separate chief dental officer who is subordinate to the Surgeon General but not the Medical Chief. In the National Institute of Health, there is a separate research institute dedicated to oral health.

In Britain, as in other parts of Europe, in particular Germany, the dental profession evolved quite differently, and as a medical speciality.

Apart from those men described earlier, who practised some form of dentistry as a sideline (dubbed The Irregulars), there were those who made dentistry their trade more or less exclusively. There were also those medically qualified men who considered dentistry an important speciality and practised it exclusively; for example, George Waite FRCS, who in 1841 described dentistry as a de facto branch of surgery, and that to be allowed to practise persons should have undergone the examinations of the Royal College of Surgeons. In 1855 he, together with seventeen other practitioners, all but four medically qualified, signed a "Memorial" to the Royal College of Surgeons asking the college to institute an examination in the department of dental surgery.

One of the Memorialists was John Tomes, 'the father of dentistry'. He was elected Fellow of the Royal Society in 1850, Honorary FRCS in 1883, and knighted in 1886. He was Dental Surgeon at the Middlesex Hospital and first President of the British Dental Association which was founded in 1879. His book, 'A Course of Lectures in Dental Physiology and Surgery', based on his histological research and wide clinical experience , laid the systematic foundations of scientific dentistry. It was a model for Fish, as indeed was Tomes' entire achievement.

In his report, "The Centenary of the First Dental Diploma in Britain", Fish writes, "There were two factions among the dentists, those who thought dentistry was a branch of surgery and those who thought it was a separate profession and should be independent. The latter actually formed a separate College of Dentists but in the end it was the former that prevailed and persuaded the Royal College of Surgeons to set up the Licence in Dental Surgery which could be awarded equally to those who were not Members of the College. (i.e. not medically qualified). It was however, the significant fact that many of those that obtained the licence were not Members that irrevocably separated dentistry from medicine.

"It therefore happened that through an error in tactics or perhaps force of circumstances, those pioneers brought about a state of affairs that was the opposite of what they intended. They wanted to make dentistry a branch of medicine, whereas in fact they established a separate profession."

It has to be remembered that until the Medical Bill of 1858 medical degrees and diplomas were granted by a hotch-potch of institutions, university faculties, the medical and surgical colleges, guilds and livery companies as well as the Society of Apothecaries. Even the Archbishop of Canterbury could grant an MD, but in 1859, Queen Victoria granted the Council of the Royal College of Surgeons, which was already an examining body in general surgery, a Royal Charter permitting them to "examine persons desirous of being so examined" and to issue certificates of fitness to practise dentistry. This did not provide the profession with autonomy. Dental surgery was now an officially recognised speciality within the general surgical framework of the College. Also, by the turn of the nineteenth century Guy's Hospital had already instituted formal lectures in dental surgery, further cementing the incorporation of dentistry within medicine.

These lectures were first given by Joseph Fox who incorporated his lectures into his books published in 1803 and

1806. Today, even though dental education has become a university discipline, its roots are reflected in its intimate relationship to the Royal College of Surgeons, and to hospital institutions.

The establishment in 1956 of the General Dental Council guaranteed a measure of autonomy to the profession, but in the eyes of many, including Sir Wilfred Fish, it had to be regarded as a speciality within medicine. It is perhaps an irony that despite this strongly held belief, one which he reiterated not long before he died, Fish played an important part in the establishment of the G.D.C.

A knighthood was conferred on Fish because of his many and various contributions to his chosen profession. By his researches into the pathology of dental diseases, and through his writings and teaching, like John Tomes before him, he forged a link between science and dental practice. Through his dedication, personality and political skills he helped regulate the profession and thereby enhanced its status.

He was a man of great integrity and independent thought, who examined and revised many traditional dental beliefs and practices, and helped to modernise the profession.

As Sir Robert Bradlaw said in his Memorial Address for Fish, "he had tenacity, intellectual honesty and humility not uncommonly found in men of like stature."

Fish brought an evangelical zeal to his profession, and his Wesleyan upbringing and education must have helped to sow the seeds of his considerable achievements.

Chapter 1

THE WESLEYAN HERITAGE

The seventeenth century saw upheaval in religious belief and practice in Britain, with fragmentation of the established Church of England, and a spectrum of faiths ranging from Roman Catholicism to Puritanism. In the middle of the eighteenth century a group of earnest Anglican students, distinguished by their devotion to piety and discipline and disillusioned with the laxity and complacency of contemporary Anglican clergy, formed a separate clerical group. It was a time when parsons were addicted to fox hunting, and when political leaders treated ecclesiastical office as a reward for party support, so that Dr.Johnson could declare that, "no man can now be made a Bishop for his learning and piety; his only chance of promotion is in his being connected with someone who has parliamentary interest." John Wesley, who had been a Fellow of Lincoln College, Oxford, and his younger brother, Charles, were leaders of this movement. They remained within the Anglican Church, and wishes to reform it from within rather than breaking away from the Mother Church. This was a point that Fish always made when writing about his background. The Wesleys and their followers came to believe that the heart of religion lies in a personal relationship with God, and in simplicity of worship. The brothers believed that the Church had a mission to save people from their sins, and the clergy were not fulfilling that mission. They pledged themselves to frequent attendance at Holy Communion and serious study of the Bible, that is to the method of worship, and to regular visits to the prisoners in the squalor of the Oxford prisons. They came to be called Methodists.

They objected to the strict hierarchical structure and practice of the Church of England, which separated ordained ministers from the laity. They were not Nonconformist in the manner of the Puritans, but bridged the divide between the latter and the Anglican Church. They established the practice of travelling the country to preach the road to salvation. John Wesley preached 'a religion of the heart', in which ritual, priestly hierarchies, and such phenomena as miracles and divine saviours played little part. This evangelical movement was set against increasing rural poverty, and it was largely, but not entirely, the poor who came to follow Wesley, and to call themselves Methodists. Some left the Church of England, but others such as William Wilberforce , the tireless campaigner against slavery, like John Wesley himself, stayed within the mother Church. It is said that John Wesley in his time, travelled a quarter of a million miles on horseback, and gave over 40,000 sermons to the godless of the Industrial Revolution, that hurricane of social turmoil that brought prosperity and despair in equal measure. He preached simplicity of worship in which laity and ministers were partners, and foremost in their concern was the plight of the underprivileged. Wesley's democratic sympathies found representation in the system of class meetings in which spiritual guidance was frequently given by laymen. The road to God did not need to be paved by stained glass windows and church ornamentation, nor was the Church and its ordained ministry an essential intermediary between Man and his Maker. Wesley gave the laity freedom to speak their mind, and in later years, not surprisingly, Methodists were to form a dedicated core, first of the Liberal Party and then of the Labour Party. Only after Wesley's death in 1795 did his followers make a formal break with the Anglican Church, and set up a Conference of a hundred men, initially clergy but subsequently to include laymen, to govern the Society of Wesleyans. The country was divided into districts, and then circuits which were groups of congregations with ministers appointed to serve the circuits. The travelling tradition remained the core of its organisation.

When Fish was born in 1894, his father, the Wesleyan minister, Reverend George Morrison Cotter Fish was on a Mission to bring the Good News of the Word of God to the people of Devon, Dorset and Somerset. There were vigorous outposts of Methodism in Ireland, and although born in Douglas, Isle of man in 1863, Fish's father was of Irish ancestry. He had found the road to salvation early in life, and at about the age of sixteen or seventeen; as Wesleyan Methodists say, "he gave himself to Christ." Almost immediately he became a local preacher, gathering the crowds of the curious and those looking for redemption, and in1886 trained in the duties of the clergy at Didsbury College. As his obituary in the Wesleyan Methodist Minutes of the Conference (1924) reads, " Zeal, wisdom and tact drew to him numbers of young men, to whom in his earlier work he became a leader in evangelistic work. He had a gracious personality, a soul fashioned for friendship, a mind furnished by habitual meditation in the best literature, and a ready tongue ruled by the law of kindness."

Before arriving with his wife Harriet at Chard in Somerset, Reverend Fish had already completed two circuits of preaching, and in Chard a son, Eric Wilfred, was born on January thirtieth 1894. He was to be the only son between two girls, Nellie and Mabel. He was baptised two months later in the Wesleyan Methodist chapel.

Chard is an ancient town of Saxon origin, sixty miles south of Bristol, and lying at the foot of the Blackdown Hills. In Reverend Fish's day it was a busy and well populated town where the manufacture of machine lace and agricultural machinery thrived. Many folk there were ripe for Methodist conversion. "Open air services woke up the people of Chard to the fact that the Methodists were in earnest to save the town." A poster announced the Mission services, and one evangelist, a Mr.Cape, took photographs and threw magic lantern images upon a large screen hung up in front of the chapel. "Dozens of people passing along the street stopped to gaze at the unusual sight, many of whom were buttoned-holed by Mrs. Fish ...".

Harriet was an ardent evangelist, and fortunately for the Fish family, not without some family means.

One daily feature of Victorian domestic life was the family at prayer, and in the household of a Wesleyan clergyman prayers would be said two or three times a day. Reading the Scriptures would certainly have been a daily habit so that the characters in the Bible became as real to the Fish children as the people around them. Bright and imaginative children have a problem in dealing with conflicting models of reality and as Fish recalled in a letter to Professor Bert Cohen, his successor as Director of Dental Science at the Royal College of Surgeons, "I gathered that the Garden of Eden was a sort of fairyland, where the snake, friendly and apparently not quite nice, talked to Eve. I was never clear why he got into such hot water for recommending her to taste the tree of knowledge, in view of the constant efforts of all around us to instil knowledge into us. But I was not sure that snakes really talked or that knowledge was easily come by." Not surprisingly, he also recalled that in his childhood "there was a constant sense of God in our home."

Darwin's "The Origin of the Species by means of Natural Selection" came out in 1859 at a time when the authority of Scripture was already being questioned, but perhaps the Reverend Fish kept such disturbing and antipathetic notions away from his children, for as Fish goes on to recall in the letter to Cohen," one night my father, a Wesleyan Minister, hearing us talking, came in with the news that Queen Victoria had died that day. I was seven and we children were quite sure that nothing could ever be the same again. Conversation in the family ranged widely over historical, political and religious subjects. Science was seldom touched on and Huxley and Darwin were not mentioned."

It seems impossible that a bright and enquiring child could have been kept away from such popular stories as Jules Verne's, "Twenty thousand leagues under the Sea" or H.G.Wells' "The Time Machine" which came out in serial form starting in 1894, the year that Fish was born. It has to be remembered that the Wesleyan creed enshrined the literal truth of the Bible story. It discouraged any other truth, and paid little attention to the rich store of the imagination in literature. However, in all his writing, Fish demonstrated a considerable debt to philosophical ideas, and often made references from the particular to these, and to general scientific ideas that would clarify and illuminate his teaching. Nevertheless, Fish always claimed that amongst his favourite reading, Storkey and Co. came first. Rudyard Kipling's tale of an anarchic, anti-establishment trio of boys, Storky, M'Turk and Beetle, which came out 1899, was so popular that it was reprinted sixteen times, and remains a model for all anti-hero stories about boys at private schools. The trio showed disrespect for their teachers, smoked in their secret hide-aways, their dialogue spiced with, 'Stinker', 'Bags I, next time' and such treasures of language as, 'Oh frabjous day! Calloo, Callay'. Their adventures must have provided an antidote to the rigours of English language lessons with their emphasis on correct use of the language, syntax and accurate spelling. What a relief, freedom of imagination was all.

By the time young Fish was sent away to Kingswood School in 1904 at the age of ten, as part of the Wesleyan system of 3-year circuits in different of different areas, the Fish family had moved on to Newark, then north to Ripon, and from there to Darlington. So many elements in the personality and work of the future Sir Wilfred can be glimpsed in his dedicated and industrious background, motivated by the Wesleyan work ethic, the credo that the road to salvation lies in making the most of every day. The injunction to "Do all the good you can, to all the people you can, in all the ways that you can, for as long as ever you can" must have been branded on his mind from an early age. Another of Fish's personality traits is revealed in a story that he told about his young self. He cut a minnow open, a large one about two inches long, he remembers, and found inside an organ which he decided was an air sac and responsible for its ability to swim, an activity he feared and hated. He was very pleased with this discovery, and says that his overwhelming feeling was to dash out and tell somebody. He just had to communicate the news. He must have listened to his father's regular preaching of a different kind of news. Later in life he commented that sometimes he broke into print or gave a lecture a bit prematurely.

Before he was sent away to school Mrs. Fish hired a governess to coach her son in Latin, which he hated, and in French, in which endeavour the governess must have succeeded because her pupil was accepted by Kingswood School.

A new century had started, one symbolised by Marconi's invention of wireless telegraphy, and by the first flight of the first motor-driven heavier than air machine by the brothers, Orville and Wilbur Wright in 1903. For some it was a time of cruel poverty, and the diseases of malnutrition such as scurvy and rickets were rife. In 1899 infant mortality reached the extraordinary figure of 163 in a 1000 births. Dental disease was so rampant that as Fish noted in his sardonic way, " As early as 1903 mincing machines were sent to the army in South Africa to supply the deficiencies in the army's dental armament."

For others it was a period of hope and opportunity, especially for the business and professional classes. Those individuals that made a personal religious commitment believed that through sobriety, discipline and character they would be set on the ladder of upward social mobility. No doubt this was in the minds of Reverend and Mrs. Fish when they sent their only son to a school with a fine scholastic reputation.

Kingswood School was founded in the eighteenth century by John Wesley for the sons of ministers, and subsequently moved into the pleasant countryside around Bath, where, now co-educational, it still prospers. In 1904 Fish along with eleven other boys entered School House. Then there were around two hundred pupils and a dozen teachers in the school. With such an enviable student-staff ratio (today at Eton it is even better at a ratio of eight to one) it was possible to provide a comprehensive curriculum taught in depth.

Most Victorian Public Schools appointed evangelical headmasters like Dr. Thomas Arnold of Rugby, and at Kingswood the ethos of the school took a Wesleyan rather than an Anglican form. The emphasis was on intellectual integrity, a spirit of moral responsibility, and on hard work. As a Wesleyan school the intimate connection between the Christian life and the faithful discharge of daily duty was strongly drilled into the pupils, many of whom went on to service in the Church, and into the educational work of the Methodist Church in India.

Mathematics was one of the school's distinctions, and many boys won awards to Oxford and Cambridge, from where many of the teachers were recruited. They were rewarded with an annual salary of One Hundred and Twenty Pounds rising to Two

Hundred Pounds after ten years. Graduates of less prestigious universities were paid on a lower scale. A teacher wanting to marry had to obtain the head's permission, and while he was resident at the school could be with his wife only at weekends.

By the year that Fish started school, football, which he disliked, had become compulsory for all boys; rugby and cricket were optional. As described in Thomas Hughes' 'Tom Brown's Schooldays', Public Schools at that time were encouraging the ethos of team games, but Fish, even then, was a reluctant team player. Out-of-school activities such as photography were encouraged, and Fish pursued this hobby with some success in later years. (One of the boys, C.E.K.Mees, went on to invent Kodachrome). Fish demonstrated his ability to draw and his sense of humour, as well as the efficiency of the Royal Mail, when at the age of thirteen he sent a letter to himself at the school with the address drawn entirely in pictograms; his name a clearly drawn denizen of the deep, the school a crown and copse of trees, and Bath, the sanitary fittings no one could mistake. The letter was delivered safely. In later years his letters to his children and grandchildren were beautifully illustrated with comic drawings.

The routine life of the school had been unchanged for many generations, Spartan, cold showers and too little food. Morning bell was at 6.20 a.m., first lesson at 7.00, and breakfast at 8.00 followed by prayers. It is recorded that, "There was morning school before breakfast. Then came the mug of tea, not too warm, and very sweet, a pat of butter the size and thickness of a couple of pennies, and a slice of bread. Too often no second slice was offered; the maids went round with shallow baskets of cut slices, and if all were taken before it reached one's seat she retired and no more came." The same fare served for tea. Fish's second wife, Hazel, Lady Fish, says that although he had a terrific sense of fun, he was not happy at school. He was forbidden to do sports because of some suspected heart problem, but later in life there was no evidence of this. Other boys played sports, Wilfred climbed trees on his own.

Lucky boys were invited once a fortnight by the Governor's wife to breakfast on cold steak and kidney pies and lashings of gravy , followed by coffee, toast and marmalade.

Although later in life Fish became a careful recorder of his research work, he left no notes of his personal life, including his school days, perhaps an indication of his misery there. The school archives tell us that there is no record of any distinction by him in sport or music, but he achieved distinction in science, for which he was awarded the school's premier Gabriel award in 1910. By this time he had passed the Oxford Local Examinations with Honours, and at the age of sixteen was therefore qualified for university entry and preparation for the life of a professional person. He obtained a further prize, and that was for 'Model Drawing' which seems to give promise of those technical skills which were to manifest themselves later in his research work and in his dental practice, except that seventy years later, in a letter to his colleague and friend, Professor Bert Cohen, Fish claimed that he never did Model Drawing and could not understand why he was given the prize.

The first Methodists had to fight to get into Oxford and Cambridge, especially if they were in the "modern" or Science Sixth". Edinburgh was the usual place for Methodist medical students to do their training, but possibly because of family in Lancashire, Fish entered Manchester University.

The eminent Anglican clergyman, Dean Inge, then eighty in 1948, wrote in a letter to Bernard Shaw, in which he comments on the quality of professional life in Edwardian times, "I do not think that anywhere in the world there has been a happier condition than that of the comfortable professional man before the two wars. Neither poverty nor riches; interesting work; a large measure of security. If we did not recognise that we were very lucky, it was our own fault."

Virginia Woolf also recalled in more romantic fashion those pre-war years as "an age of primal innocence when lovers sang like singing birds."

Chapter 2

THE BACKGROUND TO FISH'S WORK

The peripatetic lifestyle of the Fish family, and the pastoral duties of his father must have exposed the young Fish to the crippling and disfiguring manifestations of syphilis and rickets, and the wasting of tuberculosis. These diseases were rife prior to the First World War, especially in the urban areas in which the Reverend Fish preached. The flat face, saddle-nose and peg-shaped teeth of syphilis, and the bony deformities of legs and spine in rickets must have elicited the curiosity of a bright boy who, as Fish said in an interview not long before his death, had decided at an early age that he wanted to be a doctor.

Poverty and malnutrition, air pollution and dirt, were obviously powerful contributory causes to the prevalence and severity of the diseases that then abounded. In the first decade of the twentieth century over half a million people died from tuberculosis, a disease which had little respect for social class or station in life. The characters in the T.B.sanatorium of Thomas Mann's great novel, 'The Magic Mountain,' which appeared in 1924, were largely middle class. Tens of thousands of children fell victim to those contagious scourges feared by every parent, diphtheria, scarlet fever, smallpox, whooping cough and poliomyelitis. A regular sight outside some unhappy house was an ambulance into which a stretcher-borne little figure wrapped in a red blanket, was taken away to the fever hospital, all too often never to return.

As a medical student in Manchester, the most important centre of the cotton industry, Fish would have been aware of all these health problems. As a dental student he must have taken special interest in the facial and dental deformities of rickets and syphilis, as well as the dreadful oral condition of many of his patients, especially if scorbutic.

Experience of the Boer War had shown that at the end of the nineteenth century half the adult males had been found unfit for military service, and dental disease contributed substantially to that finding. Rifles were cleaned by gripping a cord between the teeth to pull it through the barrel of the gun. Those recruits who could not do this were discharged, hence the story of the rejected recruit complaining that he thought he was, "going to fight the Boers, not eat them." It was believed that "much of the failure of the man-power of the nation in the late war had its origin in this disease," that is rickets. In Paris at the turn of the century, it was estimated that 50% of children in hospital were rachitic, and it was generally believed that rickets was a disease of malnutrition. In 1914 the eminent nutritionist, Edward Mellanby, was supported by the then Medical Research Committee to study the cause of rickets, which he identified as a deficiency in a fat soluble factor, subsequently called Vitamin D. Writing in 1920 in the Lancet on the feeding of infants, Mellanby commented on the influence of diet in the differing susceptibility of Jewish and Gentile infants to rickets, "it is clear from the available dietary evidence that Jewish children received adequate anti-rachitic diets... It is likely that better maternal nutrition and the nature of the mother's diet helped to produce stronger Jewish babies, and that breast feeding practices among Jewish women contributed to reducing their infants' vulnerability to rickets."

The health situation was carefully appraised by J. Lawson Dick, when in the nineteen-twenties he was Deputy Commissioner of Medical Services, London Region. In examining the death rates of infants during the first year of life per thousand births in the years 1911-14, he noted that the figure for Shoreditch (148) was exactly twice that for the more affluent Hampstead (74), and in the second year of life it was three times as great. He concluded that " what can be attained in Hampstead ought to be attained in Shoreditch, or if that is impossible, Shoreditch should be condemned as an area unsuitable for the rearing of infant life."

These diseases were most common in the huge industrial centres such as the London Metropolitan area, and the mining centres of Durham, Yorkshire and Lancashire, and South Wales and Bristol, and in describing the background to rickets Dick writes, " The child of the slum-dweller at home lives for eighteen months-two years in the vitiated atmosphere of a close and crowded room surrounded by mean streets in the midst of a great industrial centre where all wholesome environment that makes for health is excluded." Writing after the First World War, Lawson Dick proposed that much of the failure of the man-power of the nation in that war had its origin in the high prevalence of rickets.

C.E.Wallis, who had both medical and dental qualifications, and was then assistant medical officer to the London County Council, had in 1905 carried out a systematic examination of the mouths of 245 children at the Michael Faraday school in Walworth. He found very poor oral hygiene and a great deal of oral sepsis, which he reported to the International Congress of School Hygiene.

In the same year the School Dentists' Society (which had been founded in 1899), petitioned the LCC to appoint properly qualified dental surgeons to all schools so that regular examinations and advice on prevention could be given to the children. A school dental clinic had been established in Cambridge in 1908, a development of the pioneer work of George Cunningham a decade earlier, but despite this the Council turned the petition down. However it did set up an enquiry into medical treatment for children attending elementary schools, and in 1907 reported that "the dental condition... is generally unsatisfactory ... and the more carefully the children are examined the greater the amount of disease and destruction is found."

The report continued with the statement, "with such dreadful oral conditions and the constant absorption of septic material, the chances of healthy childhood is small for lots of these infants." This was significant to Fish's research twenty years later into focal sepsis.

The LCC report also included comment on the dental health of adults. "It is known that dental caries is widespread... As a result the working capacity and even earnings of large numbers are seriously affected."

The situation in other countries was similar, and in Brussels a dental service for children had been started in 1875. A report from Germany stated that regular dental inspection showed that examination and treatment were useless unless followed by "practical measures of inculcating cleanliness among the children and by remedial treatment."

The problem of treatment remained. Dental hospitals neglected the treatment of children, and general hospitals carried out only extractions. The LCC report concluded that if left to private enterprise children would be neglected and that treatment should be provided in school clinics. But as Frederick Breese, London's first school dentist was to write many years later about dental treatment for the poverty-stricken, "To press upon the mother of a child, whose bare toes were protruding from its boots, the need for dental cleanliness with the advice to purchase a toothbrush, seemed not merely futile, but almost cruel."

By the turn of the century there had been immense improvements in public health due to transformations in drainage and sewerage, pure water supplies and street cleaning. Indeed it is fair to say that improvements in general health owed more to sanitary engineers than to doctors.

Also, by the end of the nineteenth century, great strides had been made in the germ theory of disease. Germany was where the emphasis on research and basic science started, and by 1860, with government support, numerous universities and research laboratories had been set up. By 1891 Germany had 300 scientists on medical research, while Britain had only 50, and by the end of the century research workers, mainly in Germany and France, had identified more than 20 micro-organisms associated with specific diseases. These findings brought with them greater emphasis on antisepsis and asepsis in hospital and in surgical procedures.

Research also focussed on anti-bacterial treatments that would destroy bacteria in the living body. This search for the "magic bullet" started in the laboratory of Paul Ehrlich in 1909, when he and Japanese bacteriologist, Sahachiro Hata found that an intramuscular injection of an arsenic compound could kill the syphilis causing *treponema pallidum.*

The beginning of the twentieth century also saw the growth of medical institutions throughout Europe and the USA, and increasing resources flowing in from government and private endowments. One of the most notable sources of philanthropy was set up by John D. Rockefeller in 1902. His Rockefeller Institute for Medical Research housed the first independent research laboratories in the USA, as well as funding medical schools. In Britain the Medical Research Council was set up in 1913.

The standard of living and of nutrition was rising. Cheap American wheat was arriving in Britain, and refrigerated meat from Australia and New Zealand. Bacon and eggs was regular breakfast fare for the middle classes, cheap fish and chips suppers were available to working folk. Tea, along with beer, was now the national drink, and the per capita consumption of sugar had increased from 54lbs. in 1870-99 to 85lbs. in 1900-1910.

Death rates were dropping, life expectancy for men had risen from forty to forty-four, and for women from forty-two to forty-eight.

Although large strides had been made in antisepsis, anaesthesia, both local and general, and in the organisation of the nursing profession, anything like a coherent health service was far off. Only a tiny proportion of the nation's budget was spent on health care, and of that only a small proportion was funded by the state. In 1910 only 11.2% of all medical expenditure was government funded, (that was something like £2 per person per year), while in France it was 50% more, a comparison which persisted until the start of Britain's National Health Service in 1948.

Most hospitals were founded to treat the sick poor, providing treatment for those entirely without means. There were poor law infirmaries, voluntary hospitals, and fever hospitals where wards were crowded and freezing in winter, as well as charity dispensaries. Most of these institutions depended on private philanthropy and the Charity Commissioners. Principal among these voluntary schemes was the Prince of Wales Hospital Fund established in 1897, which on Edward's accession to the throne became the King's Fund. This was set up to considerable public fanfare, to place hospitals on a sound financial footing. The Prince was against State and parochial support for hospitals and all for voluntary schemes. One interesting rider was introduced; no part of the fund should be used for medical laboratories or for medical schools which conducted experiments, "on helpless dumb animals.".

Government departments and Local Authorities vied for control of health service provision. The situation was anarchic and inadequate. Thus the eight million inhabitants of London were served by hospitals with two beds per thousand people instead of a estimated need for twice as many.

In an attempt to tackle the problems which threw many respectable people into poor law institutions, Lloyd George in 1911 introduced the National Insurance Bill and the old age pension. The Act provided insured workers with care from 'panel doctors' and access to provident and private dispensaries. This met with considerable opposition from the medical profession, many of whom believed that doctors in their beneficence should be left alone by government. Those on the left of the political spectrum, such as Beatrice Webb and the Fabian Society, proposed State employment for all doctors.

With such chaos in health care provision there had to be some sort of rapprochement between the State and the medical profession.

An influential figure at that time was the distinguished Canadian physician and professor of medicine, Sir William Osler. Earlier in his career he had carried out research at the department of physiology of University College, London where Fish was later to work. Osler played a key role in transforming the organisation and curriculum of medical education, emphasising the importance of clinical experience. In 1903 at a lecture in Oxford, he proposed that the voluntary system be ended. "Give it up", he said, " it is antiquated, out of date......you must accept the principle of taking pay from patients."

Debates about the organisation and funding of health care

provision consumed much time and energy in the early days of the century, but by 1914 such debates were interrupted by the needs of the war.

Fish's Professional Training

By 1900 there were about sixty dental schools in the USA and seven in Britain, three in London plus schools in Birmingham, Newcastle, Liverpool and Manchester.

Training at American schools was largely technical with some neglect of academic and scientific subjects. In Britain the standards required for professional qualification were set by the Royal College of Surgeons of England, the Royal Colleges of Edinburgh and of Ireland, and the Faculty of Physicians and Surgeons of Ireland. The four-year courses for the LDS diploma under the aegis of these colleges were now well established. In instituting the organisation of medical and dental schools considerable controversy arose about the relationship between clinical practitioners and scientifically based doctors. Although hospital registrars acted as tutors in medicine and surgery, a clinician with a busy private practice could not devote enough time to his subject or serve adequately as a university professor. The remedy was to institute university chairs in clinical subjects from university medical schools, and introduce academic staff into hospitals bringing together hospital wards, out-patients and laboratory facilities.

Although the sixteen-year-old Fish wanted to do medicine, his father said that he could only afford to pay for the dental course, but after two years Fish complained that the demands of the course were disappointingly too low, and that somehow money must be found for the medical course. Reverend Fish raised the necessary funds, which his son repaid as soon as he could.

When Fish started his professional training in 1910 at Manchester University the medical and dental syllabuses had evolved to the point where they formed a foundation for the teaching programmes of today, but some differences stand out.

One is the fee-paying arrangement. All courses were paid for by the term. Thus the charge for a term's lectures in physics was

£2 12s 6d while the practical physics course was £2 2s; a term's laboratory course in general chemistry held for six hours each week for the whole session from October to June cost £5 5s. The term charge for borrowing a microscope was 10s, and the dental mechanics course was charged at £4 4s per term.

These charges may seem small but when measured against the average wage of less than £100 per year, the accumulated cost of a medical or dental course was a considerable burden. One can understand the strain on their resources that Fish's parents felt as their son went through the six years needed for both courses. The stipend of a Wesleyan clergyman was not substantial.

Another manifest difference was in the employment of teaching personnel. Most medical and dental clinical lecturers and demonstrators were part-time. As Fish reported in an article written about the time of his knighthood in 1954, " there were a few short courses of lectures in Dental Metallurgy, Dental Mechanics, Dental Anatomy and practical Histology, Dental Materia Medica, and Dental Surgery - all given by part-time visiting staff. They also did clinical teaching with half-time demonstrators in Conservation and Prosthetics." The laconic, not to say dismissive tone of this account seems to indicate a less than enthusiastic respect for the standard of dental teaching he had received. In both his clinical and scientific work he was to display a considerable capacity for detailed analysis and logical thinking; to a man who set himself high standards, some of his teachers must have appeared amateur and mediocre, men who never questioned the foundations of their teaching and practise.

Vulcanite dentures and swaged metal partials, zinc oxide and eugenol dressings, gutta percha temporary fillings, grains of arsenic placed gingerly into pulp chambers to kill the pulp of infected teeth, and foot engines grindingly slow; all these will have formed the business of the student day. No matter how devoid of intellectual content all this was, as a young man who was "good with his hands" Fish would at least have enjoyed the fine detail and precision required in the mechanics laboratory. Among his fellow dental students Fish must have stood out as rather special, clever perhaps even maverick. When he put a question to one of his teachers, he was told that he was there to learn not to ask questions. But as he said, " a deeply ingrained attitude of mind has been with me from childhood. When I read or was told how to do something I often asked, 'Why?' and often, 'Why not some other way?'"

Apparently at a very tender age he cut open his mother's bellows to see where the air came from. Fish said that his mother was very upset but didn't punish him. She must have been very indulgent to her only son. Later, as his father was hopeless in practical matters the young Fish would mend punctures on his father's bicycle.

Fish's account of a viva on periodontology is illuminating. "The extent of dental knowledge when I took my Final LDS in 1914 on this subject was well illustrated by a question in my viva. One examiner asked me whether pyorrhoea caused tartar or did tartar cause pyorrhoea? I caught the glint in the other examiner's eye. 'Well sir,' I said, ' There are some say one thing and some say the other.' 'What did I tell you,' said my examiner to his colleague, giving him a dig in his ribs with his elbow, and they both laughed and dropped the subject. Nevertheless I thought it well worth investigating the matter when I had the time."

And time was to prove him right.

Students have always been perceptive critics of their teachers, and while some of Fish's teachers must have been the subject of student's jokes, at least two of the full-time staff engaged in teaching pre-clinical subjects in Manchester at that time were men of extraordinary achievement.

The head of the physics department was Ernest Rutherford, the father of atomic physics and winner in 1908 of the Nobel prize. Fish regarded Rutherford with reverence; if Fish ever had a hero it was Rutherford. Indeed it is impossible to imagine that first year students like Fish were not overwhelmed by the presence of this huge rugby playing man with the rough accent of rural New Zealand, described as a "great booming bear", whose work led to the modern understanding of the atom. Before Rutherford the atom had been regarded as the ultimate particle of which all else was made, and solid as a ball-bearing. Rutherford showed that the atom was largely empty space, with at its centre, a tiny nucleus. He was a prodigious worker with remarkable powers of concentration, who wrote eighty scientific papers during his seven years teaching at McGill University before he was invited to a chair at Manchester. Later in life in talks to various groups, Fish would describe Rutherford's work at the Cavendish Laboratory at Cambridge, where he discovered a magnetic detector of electro-magnetic waves which could signal through a half-mile of brick walls and houses, and the day that Rutherford announced, holding up a negative, "Gentlemen. I am afraid that we have split the atom"

It is unlikely that Fish, unless he actually visited Rutherford's laboratory, encountered Rutherford's research assistant, who with Rutherford designed an apparatus that could count particles as they were emitted from radium atoms. This radiation detection unit with its audible clicking counter bears the name of that assistant, Hans Geiger.

After working with Rutherford, Geiger returned to Germany to become an ardent supporter of Hitler. He was one of the most active of senior scientists to support the Nazis. He turned against his Jewish colleagues, including those who had helped in his career, and refused all help in their requests to find posts out of Germany. It is therefore improbable that he had much to do with Fish's lecturer in organic chemistry, Chaim Azriel Weizmann.

Weizmann who was born in Motol, a hamlet in Western Russia, the third of fifteen children of orthodox Jewish parents, was destined to become in 1948 the first President of the new State of Israel. After taking a doctorate he taught chemistry in Geneva before taking up his appointment at Manchester University in 1904. He gained influence for the Zionist cause by his political activity, and also by giving valuable assistance to the munitions industry in the Great War. In 1916 the industry was in dire need of acetone, a vital ingredient of the smokeless explosive cordite. Weizmann devised a method of extracting acetone from maize, an achievement which helped the Zionists who were then negotiating with the British government about the return of the Jews to Palestine. In 1917 Arthur Balfour, then Foreign

Secretary, made the famous Declaration naming Palestine as a homeland for the Jews.

There is no evidence that until he arrived in Manchester that Fish had any contact with Jewish people, except for the Biblical characters of his youth. But by the beginning of the century Manchester had a sizeable Jewish community, and many of Fish's patients at both the dental school and at Manchester's General Hospital, must have been Jewish. One can imagine that his later sympathy with those doctors and dentists who fled Nazi persecution in the nineteen-thirties to seek asylum in Britain, might have had some connection with his teacher in organic chemistry.

There were slight differences in the university degree courses for the BDS and the diploma course for LDS. While many of the pre-clinical courses were attended by LDS, BDS and MB students together, the pathology and bacteriology course for LDS was less detailed. Many medical and dental students took the "conjoint" examinations, that is those for the diplomas given by the Royal Colleges, because these were believed to be easier than the examinations for university degrees.

Fish qualified as a dental surgeon in 1914 with an LDS diploma, and apparently then, he and his fellow student, H.H.Stones, had some difficulty negotiating their entrance to the university examinations for the MB, ChB rather than the diplomas MRCP, LRCS. The Dean, Mr. Hilditch Mattthews, reported that Messrs. E.W.Fish and H.H.Stones (who was to become the Dean of the Liverpool Dental School) had entered the MB course without permission. This in no way prejudiced Fish's undergraduate career. Before he qualified in medicine he was appointed to a junior Resident post at Salford Royal Hospital and then recommended for a Resident appointment. In the final MB ChB examinations in 1916, a year after Stones qualified, Fish was awarded the Dumville Surgical Prize, value £15 to be spent on books or instruments. He was described as an excellent anaesthetist and a careful and dependable worker.

The Dental Register shows that Fish was first registered LDS in February 1915, and MB ChB in 1917, by which time he was in the army. Soon after Fish had obtained his dental diploma he was called up, and in June 1915 as Lieutenant Fish was appointed Dental Surgeon to the 2nd. Western General Hospital in Manchester, his assignment to examine and where necessary provide dental treatment to wounded soldiers in hospitals in that area. The letter from his commander to "all concerned" was that they "are requested to kindly afford every facility to Lieutenant Fish." His address in 1915 is given as 140 Manchester Road, Bury, which continued to be his address until 1920.

In 1916, the second year of the Great War, the army's hope that the voluntary system of recruitment would provide sufficient manpower faded and a new scheme of recruitment, that is conscription, was put in place.

In July 1917, now doubly qualified and a married man, Captain Fish was assigned to the Bombay Regiment, 6th. Poona Division, as temporary Specialist in Advanced Operative Surgery. The year before Fish had married Hilda Gertrude Russell, whose father Samuel Joseph Russell had been a chartered accountant until, as his obituary records, " he heard the call of God to the Ministry of the Methodist Church in Canada" where he did pioneer work among the cod fishermen and backwoodsmen of Labrador. In 1902 he returned to England and spent most of his ministry in the industrial centres of the North. Presumably this is how one of Fish's sisters met the minister's daughter, Hilda Gertrude, and introduced her to her brother Wilfred. His sister Mabel had a degree in music and played the piano, and one can imagine the high spirits of these young people when the war was over. Nellie, the elder sister, married a contemporary of her brother's at dental school, E.V. Pollitt, who became a local authority dental officer in Lancashire. They kept in touch all their lives, and occasionally Fish would send Pollitt drafts of his papers for comment. Mabel made a rather turbulent marriage, and emigrated to America. According to Lady Fish they were a family of great character. The story goes that Miss Russell took one kiss as a sign that she and Fish were engaged. Fish's future was sealed, and marriage became inevitable. After Hilda's father, Reverend Russell, retired he went to live in

Sevenoaks in Kent where after the war Fish had started in dental practice.

Fish was a man who, at least for the record, rarely talked or wrote about his personal life to his colleagues. He kept his personal and professional lives quite separate. Molly Goulding, his secretary for many years at a time when he had already achieved considerable success, recalled that he never mentioned his first wife and their family, or his time in war service. But he did keep a hand-written memoir of his time in the army from when he enlisted with the Bombay Brigade.

In 1903 the Bombay Brigade had become a pioneer unit, that is, as well as being a fully trained infantry unit it was also trained in technical work such as road and railway building, and in mining and sapping. It was engaged in the disastrous Mesopotamian campaign against the Turks, as well as in Egypt and Palestine. Any engagements in India were mainly on the Afghanistan front, the North West frontier, where tribal rebellions took place in the hill country near Peshawar.

Fish is named in the Indian Army List as a specialist in advanced operative surgery at Kolaba, which is a district of Bombay, where he worked at a base hospital treating head and maxillo-facial wounds. Official records make no mention of his work or time in India, but the memoir of this period in his life is very revealing.

Fish divided this record of his time in the army into ten chapters starting with his enlistment in Blackpool, Lancashire being his home then, travelling from there to Marseilles, and then sailing on the troopship Cameronia to Malta. The journey from there to Egypt is intriguingly entitled 'Further Facts and Fictions', an extraordinarily cool title for the events described. In writing this account it is possible that Fish was influenced by the story published in 1913, of Captain Scott's tragic second expedition to the South Pole, and especially by Captain Lawrence Oates' last words knowing he was going to his death, "I am going outside and may be some time." These few words must have imprinted themselves on all their readers as a model of how an English gentleman should behave.

The Times of India reported that on the 15th. April 1917 the troopship Cameronia was hit by a torpedo in the afternoon on a calm sea. The submarine was invisible. The explosion was severe and killed and injured many of the crew and soldiers, British, Scottish and Irish but mostly men from the Midlands. In his version of events Fish writes, "It was not a loud noise as explosions go. There was no deafening crash and yet that subdued determined thud, the quiver of the ship like a wounded animal, the acrid smell of T.N.T. removed the suspicion that a steward had stepped on a stair that wasn't there with a tray of dishes in his hand.... With a cool and steady step we hurried from the saloon to the boat deck... there on the sloping deck we worked, white faced but determined."

Fish describes the chaos of trying to get soldiers into the boats; "the first boat launched was smashed with many casualties..... The Chief Officer perished while diving in an attempt to rescue a soldier who had fallen between the ships." Men were running from one deck to another to reach the boats being lowered from the sinking ship, but when ordered, "'from here to the right get back on deck' the boys responded at once, not a murmur, not a look behind, and the boats were swung out. Soon the sea was dotted with boats and rafts while the (rescuing) destroyers steamed around like angry dogs." The Cameronia sank in thirty-five minutes, and because there were no more boats, Fish spent part of that time in the water, finally succeeding in grabbing a rope to be pulled to safety on board one of the destroyers.

After a brief stay in Egypt his regiment moved on to India which was reached safely. There Fish set to work at the Colaba Hospital on a regular hospital routine of operations including general surgery, a routine that was to be interrupted by a severe bout of dysentery which kept him in hospital as a reluctant patient for several weeks.

According to Lady Fish her husband enjoyed that interesting immunological phenomenon, dermographism, in which the sufferer can write on his skin because red wheals are raised in the skin under pressure. Fish felt so ill that he wrote 'DEATH' on his chest. His memoir records this episode as 'A trying experience.'

He was sent to convalesce at a village called Nasik, high in the hills above Bombay, where he was able to stroll around and observe the exotic plants and native customs. He noted that "very few women were to be seen, and those who were abroad, tho' quite unconscious of any immodesty of exposing generous quantities of thigh and leg, were careful to so cover their head and shoulders as only to leave a narrow slit for their eyes..."

He had hoped to be allowed back to work at the hospital, but was judged not fit enough and sent home. He travelled with a letter from his immediate superior, Major Norman McLaren, Commander of the Colaba War Hospital, stating that Captain Fish had special experience of the surgery of the mouth and face, and was best fitted for surgical work in a general hospital. Fellow officers added their comments. " A good officer who has carried out his dental and surgical work satisfactorily." "He has done good work." And even more briefly his colonel, who probably did not know him well, "I concur." Fish had been on active service in India for under a year.

As the returning ship approached Plymouth in February 1918 Fish made a final sad and enigmatic entry in his notebook. "Here I will close this record almost without apology for those for whom it is written ought to appreciate the fierce amount of exertion it has cost, and those for whom it is not should not be reading it - The rest won't."

His personal experiences, crowded into such a short time, being torpedoed and rescued from the water, his illness and the unpleasant treatment of the time for dysentery, plus his experiences as a novice surgeon, aged 23, operating on the severely wounded, about whom he makes no mention, must have been extremely distressing. There are occasional flashes of humour in these records, but for a man of such impish humour their rarity testifies to this harrowing period of his life. Although one of his practice assistants later in life described Fish as austere, as Lady Fish and many of those with whom he worked, testify, his sense of humour seems to have been readily stimulated. Maybe that assistant did not come up to expectations.

Years later Fish did tell Professor Bert Cohen, his colleague at the Royal College of Surgeons, that his ship had been torpedoed on the way to India, but it seems he treated the episode very lightly. Nor did he say, in the manner of the unflappable English gentleman, that he was the last man to be rescued as he helped his shipmates to be pulled out of the sea.

Even that early in the century German submarines represented a serious threat to Allied shipping, as they were to be 25 years later. In the year 1916 the submarine U-35 sank 54 merchant ships, and a troopship on its way to Salonika was sunk with the loss of 930 soldiers. Initially hospital ships were brilliantly lit and carried a large red cross, a perfect target for German torpedoes, but from 1917 the red cross was painted out.

By the First World War maxillo-facial surgical techniques had reached a stage of relative sophistication. Chloroform anaesthesia was used, prophylactic tetanus injections were given, but blood transfusion was not practised. Good drainage of the wounds was essential. Saline injections, warmth, lots of hot drinks and sleep "served to restore a man", Eusol was the routine antiseptic. In India high temperature and humidity led to dehydration, and flies landing on wounds to infection. For jaw injuries cap splints of tin or vulcanite were ligatured in position.

In Macpherson's 'Surgery of the War', produced in 1922 as a government document, there is a section on "Injuries to Face and Jaw" written by a B. Mendleson, LDS RCS Eng., Captain Dental Surgeon. He writes:-

"It is particularly essential in the early stages to render the buccal cavity as clean as possible. Roots, carious teeth and foreign bodies should be removed, the remaining teeth scaled, constant irrigation of the mouth practised and teeth and gums painted with iodine and picric solution. By such measures sepsis is checked, healing accelerated and septic pneumonia inhibited".

Of the British and Empire troops who had served in the war, almost a million had been killed in action and two million wounded. Total Allied dead amounted to five million men, the French losing 1,400,000 and the Russians 1,700,000. The enemy forces lost 3,500,000 of which almost 1,800,000 were German. Almost every European town and village had its war memorial.

After the war almost one million war pensions were being paid out to the British injured, gassed, blinded and shell-shocked.

By the end of the war there was growing realisation that much disease was preventable, and that the best means of preserving health and curing disease should be "available to all as a right rather than by favour."

In 1919 the Ministry of Health was created. Many specialist hospitals were founded, such as the Hospital for Tropical Diseases and St. Thomas's Babies' Hospital. Postgraduate medical training, which had started at the beginning of the century, was formalised. After 1918 it became clear that any medical or dental school that was to enjoy a place in the frontline of teaching must conform to the requirements of the University Grants Commission to obtain a grant as a school of a university. The planks were being nailed into place for today's education in medicine and dentistry, and for an organised health service.

It was a world in which those doctors and dentists who were lucky enough to have survived the war, could see a future laid out rather more clearly than before. In 1921 in response to an obvious need for more dentists, under the 1921 Dental Act, the Dental Register was opened up to practitioners without formal qualifications.

In that year Fish entered the Dental and Electoral Registers as at Buckhurst Lodge, Sevenoaks, Kent, and like all healthy ex-servicemen, despite a looming economic depression, he was ready to give the future his best shot. As Siegfried Sassoon wrote about his feelings on being demobilised in 1919, "I was in a ferment of post-war emotional release." One can imagine Sassoon's words applying to Fish on leaving the army, a married man, soon to be a father, and determined to make the best use of his talents and his war-time experiences.

In that year in the wider world the Covenant of the League of Nations was being negotiated, its aspirations to be utterly undermined by the Treaty of Versailles, which despite opposition, imposed grossly unfair territorial and economic conditions on the defeated Germans. Nobody, not even the great economist J.M. Keynes, whose writings condemned the treaty, could have predicted that the treaty would spawn the consequent rise of Hitler and the Nazi regime, a calamity that would throw Europe into yet another and even more horrific conflict.

Chapter 3

MAKING A START

Following the catastrophe of the Great War rebuilding the normal pattern of peacetime life got off to an uncertain start. As Asa Briggs points out in his 'Social History of England', "the psychological gap between 'civvy street' and the soldiers' war was far wider between 1914 and 1918 than it was to be during the 'people's war' of 1939 to 1945". The Second war was one of mobility and openness where officers and other ranks mixed to a much greater degree than in the trenches of the previous war. Also the widespread bombing of the Second war involved the whole civilian population in a way quite unknown in the First war. That war had drained the people and the economy. Before 1914 Britain was still the largest trading nation and merchant marine power, but had lost her position to the USA as leader of the world's industrial power. There was an homogeneous working class culture rooted in the common experience of mass production. Britain was a class-ridden society. For many workers in Britain, the 1917 Bolshevik revolution in Russia was regarded as a harbinger of things to come, to some an ominous threat, but for other folk a political miracle promising better times. Attitude to the revolution was one factor that promoted considerable industrial unrest in Britain, as well as dividing the wartime coalition Cabinet. Even the king, George V, feared that revolution could happen in Britain, especially during the great strikes of the following years. The Labour Party dropped out of the government, and in the General Election of December 1918, Lloyd George's next coalition government gained a resounding vote of confidence, but that confidence was destined to be short lived. The post-war boom began well enough but it was very patchy, as was the success of Lloyd George's 'reconstruction' government. The Representation of the People Act of 1918 guaranteed for the first time something like genuine democracy. It gave the franchise to women householders and wives of householders over the age of thirty. The political scene was set for the Labour Party to be the main party of opposition, and then in 1924 to form a minority government, with the former pacifist, Ramsay MacDonald, as Prime Minister. Fish, according to Hazel, was if anything a Liberal and became a member of the Liberal Club, which is not surprising considering his Wesleyan Methodist upbringing. The moral earnestness of Gladstone had attracted Nonconformists to the Liberal cause, and it was with their continuing support that the Liberal Lord Rosebury succeeded Gladstone as Prime Minister in 1894, the year that Fish was born.

Following 1918, in many parts of Britain , in particular those of our traditional major industries, coal mining, steel and ship-building which were in decline, there was considerable unemployment and unrest. Poverty in Britain was widespread, even in the midst of plenty, but the better-off, especially in the south of England, were scarcely aware of these difficulties, and if they were, were often unconcerned. Such social events as Ascot and the Henley Regatta continued uninterrupted. Any social cohesion brought about by the common objectives of fighting and winning the war was quickly replaced by the resurgence of individualism and the drive to achieve personal fulfilment. The energy and talent of the individual was needed to build post-war Britain, and the young Fish was part of that drive.

Revolutions in science had already taken place. Einstein's theories had shattered Newtonian principles that gave a rational structure to the universe, and Rutherford, Fish's former physics teacher at Manchester, had predicted the splitting of the atom.

And at a more deeply personal level, Freud's theories had shaken ideas about the mind and our unconscious drives. It was a time of scientific excitement, political and social turbulence, as well as changes in the moral climate. Personal religious commitment with its integrity and sobriety, which had formerly been a help to upward social mobility, was becoming out-of-date.

The Great War had brought about a relaxation in social attitudes of all sorts; firmly held ideas about temperance, the sanctity of the Sabbath, and hostility to the established Church had diminished. Also the non-conformist churches, unlike the Anglican Church, depended upon the economics of the local community, traditionally the miners, agricultural and textile workers. When in times of depression these industries suffered, support for the non-conformist churches faded and non-conformist values were weakened. These values coincided with those of the Liberal Party, and it was no accident that this time saw the waning of the Liberal Party with the Labour Party taking its place as a party of power and the main opposition to the Conservatives.

If not earlier, something of Fish's Wesleyan upbringing must have been undermined through the war, for both Lady Hazel Fish and Molly Goulding, his secretary of some thirty years later, testify to his complete lack of interest in formal religion. Nevertheless the Wesleyan work ethic dominated his life from the day he started his dental practice in Sevenoaks in Kent.

With its rich soil and favourable climate, as well as its proximity to the markets of London, Kent has been rightly called the Garden of England. For centuries its agriculture enjoyed prosperity, and with the coming of the railways towards the end of the nineteenth century, towns like Tonbridge, Tunbridge Wells and Sevenoaks became part of the commuter belt around London.

When the fast train from Cannon Street station took only 29 minutes to reach Sevenoaks, City gents, stockbrokers, bankers, directors of the insurance industry, and successful engineers, all and sundry in their striped suits, bowler hats and tightly rolled umbrellas, were able to travel daily between their offices and splendid houses set in large well tended gardens. They constituted a potential clientele for any up-and-coming professional man.

On demobilisation Fish went to work at Sidcup Hospital with J.F.Colyer who had worked there and at Croydon Hospital from 1914. Colyer was one of the pioneers who, mainly through their experience in the treatment of jaw fractures, were able to collaborate with plastic surgeons and devise techniques for the repair of wounds to the head and face. In 1920 he was to be knighted for his 'substantial services' in the war.

In 1893 when he was only twenty-seven Colyer had been the co-author with Morton Smale, sometime Dean of the Royal Dental Hospital, of the book, 'Diseases and Injuries of the Teeth'. In its nine editions, this was to be one of the most important dental texts. In 1910, Colyer changed the title to 'Dental Surgery and Pathology', and wrote the later editions jointly with another important figure, Evelyn Sprawson.

From 1900 Colyer served as curator of the Odontological Museum at the Royal College of Surgeons for the next 54 years, and donated 2,600 skull specimens from his collection. He also served as Dean of the Royal Dental Hospital from 1904 to 1909, and when Fish joined him at Sidcup Hospital, Colyer was one of the most eminent men in the profession.

It must have been immensely encouraging for Fish , then twenty-six and about half Colyer's age, to work with the great man. Colyer, like all dental teachers of his time, had a thriving private practice in the heart of London's medical district at 10 Queen Anne Street, and was a consultant to both Charing Cross Hospital and the nearby Royal Dental Hospital in Leicester Square. It is very likely that Colyer presented a model to which Fish could aspire, and as Molly Goulding, describes him, he was a very focussed man; focussed on his profession, and not really interested in world affairs.

Even though it is likely that Fish would have agreed with the Prime Minister of France, Clemenceau's declared policy "weaken and destroy Germany in every possible way", it is unlikely that he took much interest in the international wrangling over the terms of the 1919 Treaty of Versailles. Was he aware of the fact that in Italy by 1921 Mussolini was making Fascism into a significant political force? As with most people in Britain at that time, it seems doubtful, but following his army service in India, Fish must have taken an interest in the protests against British rule in India and Gandhi's non-cooperation movement, which had started by that time.

Any religious belief was replaced by his dedication to personal success; what of Methodism remained was his sense of purpose, the belief that salvation lay in making the most of every day, the call to action, and like his evangelist parents the demands of his own particular crusade.

After the war he must have contemplated a career in medicine, which had been his first choice, an aspiration since childhood, but in medicine the possession of a dental qualification gave little if any advantage, while in the dental profession a medical qualification almost guaranteed a secure future and access to the higher realms of the profession. After Fish retired he made notes reflecting on his work in dentistry, in particular his studies of dentine and bone, and on vitamins, and mused," Looked at as a whole, this series of experiments did make filling a tooth an intelligent and intelligible operation as far as I am concerned and if I hadn't done it I am pretty sure I should have switched into surgery - either general or specialized, in some other, better understood field."

Keen to make a reputation and earn a decent living, Fish followed Colyer's recommendation to work in Sevenoaks, and there Fish lived and practised for almost twenty years. Sevenoaks is scarcely twenty miles from Sidcup, and a pleasant and prosperous place to live and run a practice. Kent's agriculture prospered. It had escaped much of the upheaval of the industrial revolution, and its acres of fruit trees and hops laid out in neat patches of land, would have seemed like paradise to a man recently returned from India. It is not surprising that in 1921 Winston Churchill, who later became a patient of Fish's, initially at the Sevenoaks practice, bought Chartwell Manor in Kent, despite the fact that it needed almost rebuilding, and his wife, Clementine, thought it far too big and beyond their means.

That was the year that after the short-lived post-war economic boom, The Economist called, "one of the worst years of depression since the industrial revolution."

Nevertheless the South East remained relatively prosperous, especially for the middle classes. Infant mortality is a good guide to the general health, and social and economic condition of a population. Although this was dropping generally, the differential between that for the professional class compared with the unskilled in the South East was 63%, whereas the differential mortality between the classes in Lancashire and Cheshire was 198%.

At this time one of the rough demarcations between the working and middle classes was the earning figure of £250 per year. This was where the middle class was reckoned to begin and the working class ended. However many people such as clerks and salesmen, today's 'white-collar workers', who earned less than that, thought of themselves, and were regarded by those below as middle class.

Fish now belonged to the comfortable world of the professional person in Southern England, so different from the peripatetic and pious life of his parents, moving as they did among the poor of the northern counties. He recognised the potential of Sevenoaks; apart from being a pleasant town where property prices were reasonable, the town had few dentists and plenty of people who could afford good dentistry. It was not far from London, but was sufficiently rural for him to live a country-style life and indulge in his favourite pastime, horse riding. He seemed to fit into the community very well. As a personable young man, who had survived the war in which he had served as a surgeon, he was well received, and the fact that he was assisting a distinguished surgical knight at a local hospital was sufficient in itself to warrant recognition and respect. He was also immensely energetic, self-confident and ambitious.

Although not the product of a major public school he had been very well educated at a well regarded establishment, and was readily accepted by the burghers of the town, whose aspirations were like his, for material well-being and status. After all, affluence meant success.

Unlike in the aftermath of the Second World War when the class structure of Britain was seriously questioned, the return to peace in 1918 meant a return to traditional social forms and attitudes. The well-off middle class folk who came to form the core of Fish's practice were very conscious of their own and their neighbour's position in the social hierarchy. As Agatha Christie was to remark through the mouth of her Belgian detective, Hercule Poirot, dentistry was regarded as a humble profession, a craft where manual skills were necessary rather than brain power, certainly on a lower rung than medicine. Prior to 1921 many if not most dentists had no professional qualification. Their training had been by apprenticeship, and the line between dentist and dental technician was hazy.

During the war the government woke up to the fact that, as Norman Bennett, then Chairman of the BDA Council, said, " the condition of the teeth of the nation was horrible, and that a healthy and efficient people could not exist with bad teeth." The obvious need for more dentists led to the institution of the Dentists Act of 1921 and the formation of a Dental Register of all those qualified to practise, either by formal qualification or by long experience in respected practice.

Therefore, after the Act there were three classes of dental practitioner; the so-called "1921 men", those men with a dental diploma or degree, and those practitioners with both medical and dental qualifications. The latter were the elite of the profession from whose ranks most dental teachers and hospital dental surgeons or "honoraries" were drawn. This elite was few in number in Kent at a time when the urban population was increasing in number and growing in prosperity.

However the social position of those men who were qualified in both medicine and dentistry was anomalous; although equal in training to their colleagues who practised medicine, those who practised dentistry were definitely not perceived as equal in their role as health professionals. Dental health was not well valued.

Fish confounded the pattern because although he continued to practise dentistry, once he had gained his MD, he possessed a medical qualification superior to that of most doctors around him. He was not simply regarded as a "good dentist" he was obviously unique in that part of the world. Indeed a survey of the Dental Register of that time shows that he was almost singular. Many of his colleagues as Honorary Dental Surgeons to general hospitals where they carried out oral surgery, acquired an FRCS, but of his contemporaries only F.C.Wilkinson, MD 1917, who in 1924 aged thirty-five, was appointed to the newly created Chair of Dental Science at the University of Melbourne, was so well qualified.

As someone very special, Fish was in demand by those who wanted and could afford to pay for the best, and in the aftermath of the war South East England provided many of them, and once Fish's practice had grown to the point where he took on assistants, they were the ones who carried out the run-of-the-mill dentistry.

Although the National Insurance Act of 1911 allowed Approved Societies to provide dental treatment "if they had surplus funds", the first State dental benefits paid only part of the cost of treatment to render a patient dentally fit. Treatment was limited to workers earning less than a certain amount, with membership longer than about two years. This support was not available before the age of seventeen so that 14-year old school-leavers had no treatment for three years after school. Even with this limited provision, uptake was poor, partly from fear of the dentist, partly from apathy and lack of appreciation of the benefits of dental health. It is possible that in the early days of his practice Fish treated patients under these terms, but it is more than likely that very soon all his patients were treated privately.

As in all other occupations, no matter how well qualified one might be, it always takes time to prove one's self in practise, and dentistry is no exception; extractions have to be painless, fillings to stay in, and dentures provide comfortable and efficient eating machines. In 1920 Fish set up home at 1 Park Lane, close to the north end of the Vine Cricket Club pitch. His practice was not far away, but nearer the centre of Sevenoaks at 154 High Street, an old building on a prominent corner site. In that year his first child, a daughter Vivien, was born, providing a further incentive for hard work and a secure income. Soon after he moved to more permanent addresses, practising at Buckhurst Lodge until 1930, with his home nearby at 'Corona', Granville Road.

Indeed all his addresses until 1939, when he sold the practice and departed Sevenoaks for central London, were in the same pleasant, leafy part of the town.

Success and a good income does not come overnight, and as a young man starting his practice, Fish made furniture for his home, an activity for which he had a real talent. H.A.Harris, who was to become Professor of Anatomy at University College and then at Cambridge, was a senior demonstrator in the physiology department at University College when Fish as an Honorary Research Assistant, carried out the research for his MD, tells the story that when he stayed at Fish's home he admired some furniture and was informed that it had been made by his host. Next morning, not knowing what time breakfast was to be served, Harris rose early to find Fish already in his workshop, and when Harris apologised for getting Fish up so early, Fish replied that he had already been up for a couple of hours working on a table. "I never sleep for long," he said. As Professor A.E.W. (Loma) Miles, one of Fish's students at the Royal Dental Hospital, who became a junior colleague, recalls, "Fish was one of those people who need little sleep, always restless to make good use of what time he had."

Fish confirmed Miles' judgement by registering for an MD at Manchester University and starting on the research for his thesis at about the time he started his dental practice. He ran the two activities concurrently and virtually as two full-time occupations. Indeed this seems to have been the pattern of his working life.

It was commonplace for him to discuss his research late into the night, and his daughter, Vivien, remembers him at home working at his microscope into the small hours. Fortunately he was very fit and took to riding every morning before the working day. Lady Fish says that he was quite athletic and a very good oarsman, which he demonstrated on their honeymoon at Lake Como. But his passion was a sport of the upper classes, deer stalking in Ireland.

The MD Research

At the beginning of the century cocaine was used as a local anaesthetic, but its side-effects were many and occasionally fatal. It was largely discarded when the much safer drug Procaine, was synthesised in 1905 by Alfred Eishorn. One of the problems with such anaesthetic solutions was their rapid dispersion in the bloodstream which limited the period of effective anaesthesia. To prolong this period adrenaline chloride was added to the solution.

This reduced the blood flow in the area, slowed the absorption of procaine into the bloodstream so reducing its toxicity, and produced a relatively bloodless operative field. These advantages were quickly recognised and use of the combined solutions became routine practise.

In a note that Fish wrote in May 1971 about the research for his MD thesis he states, "At that time every few weeks there was reported a death in the dental chair due to injection of local anaesthetic solution. One of these (I think "Crown") contained 1% Cocaine in 1/1000 Adrenaline."

At the time of Fish's researches the minutes of hospital medical committees recorded with unhappy frequency fatalities associated with both general and local anaesthesia . Chloroform and cocaine were largely responsible. Deaths might have been even more common, but the Dangerous Drugs Act of 1921 limited dentists to the prescription of drugs "for local use only". Feeling faint and syncope were the most common side-effects of local anaesthesia, and as a practitioner with by now considerable experience of giving these injections, Fish was intrigued by this problem. In the introduction to his MD thesis, Fish notes that the addition of adrenaline produced transient feelings of faintness in 6% of his recorded cases after injection with as little as 1 in 70,000 adrenaline. He adds, "Less frequently the patient became very pale and tremulous, the pulse was small and rapid or imperceptible. Respiration was shallow and loss of consciousness sometimes supervened." The frequency and degree of collapse appeared directly related to the presence and concentration of adrenaline. It was also recognised that some people, especially women and children, and those with impaired cardiac function suffered these symptoms more frequently and severely.

These observations formed the background to Fish's research into the "Cardio-vascular effects of local anaesthetic injections (with special reference to the Effects of Adrenaline)", the subject of his thesis.

At that time Fish had no formal connection with an institution with research facilities, but the physiology department at

University College offered facilities to "Persons who are desirous of conducting original investigations in physiology and histology". The fees were comparatively small; a registration fee of One Pound Eleven Shillings and Sixpence, and a laboratory fee of Five Guineas. The opportunity was there and characteristically Fish took it. Fortunately there was a regular express train service between Sevenoaks and Charing Cross station.

The facilities of the physiology department allowed him to use cats and dogs as experimental animals. He studied the effects of various injection solutions, cocaine and procaine (Novocaine), with and without varying concentrations of adrenaline on healthy animals and on those with artificially impaired cardiac function. In the attempt to explain the variation in cardiac response to the drugs, Fish used six parameters of heart activity: blood pressure, mean heart volume, pulse rate, amplitude of contraction at each systole, output of the heart and work of the heart per unit of time.

The experimental procedure followed that of the rather inelegant but routine methods of physiological research at that time, and was much more gross than most dental research. Under general anaesthesia, and with artificial respiration administered through a tracheal cannula, a variety of injection materials were delivered through a cannula in the jugular vein. A third cannula in the femoral artery and connected to a manometer recorded blood pressure. The thorax was opened to permit a cardiometer connected to a piston recorder, to be placed directly on the heart. This showed changes in heart volume. The technique for impairing cardiac function was to tie ligatures onto the mitral valve to keep it open.

Fish found that "when a full dose of Novocaine, without any other drug, was injected in a 2% solution, no effect was observed on the circulation. When however a small dose of adrenaline was added …. the effect was much more marked. Blood pressure rose, heart volume increased, pulse rate rose (briefly), amplitude of heart beat per unit of time increased 30% and the work done per unit of time increased 80%".

In a series of graphs Fish was able to explain the variation in effects of varying doses of adrenaline in a variety of proprietary anaesthetic solutions on the healthy and impaired heart.

His conclusions in summary were that adrenaline should be used in dilutions of 1:70,000 -1:100,000; that it must not be injected into a vein, and that it must be avoided in patients with heart disease.

The year 1924 was a very rewarding one; Fish's second child, a son James Morrison Russell, was born on the 6th. January, and Manchester University awarded Fish an MD for his thesis. In the same year, the thesis was published in the British Dental Journal , but if Fish had anticipated enthusiastic comment, he must have been disappointed. The only letter published was written by F.N. Doubleday from Guy's Hospital. He was gracious enough to write that this "is the type of research we all desire to see", but he went on to comment that all Fish's injections were into veins, but in clinical practice injection is into connective tissue, therefore "the experimental conditions under which these observations were based, insufficiently resembled those under which local anaesthetics are administered in practice".

Doubleday goes on to hope that "we should aim at a steady reduction and eventual elimination of this drug (adrenaline) in local anaesthetic solutions."

As we know this hope was not to be fulfilled; sixty years later adrenaline at 1 in 80,000 is routinely used universally.

Doubleday went on to carry out a curious investigation that he reported the following year to the Section of Odontology of the Royal Society of Medicine. He studied the effects of various chemical substances including local anaesthetic solutions, on the heart muscle of decerebrated frogs, and concluded, " The results are in contradiction to those various writers who have reported that adrenaline produces an increased contraction of heart muscle. It is suggested that adrenaline has a directly depressing action on the nerve-endings and muscle fibres of the heart."

At that meeting the President of the Odontological Section was Douglas Gabell, an honorary dental surgeon at the Royal Dental Hospital, whose staff Fish was soon to join. Gabell was to become a good and supportive friend.

Coincident with this work for his MD, Fish was using the facilities of U.C.L's physiology department laboratory for quite different research on a very different scale. Physically that scale was much smaller, but its impact on Fish's career was possibly greater. It concerned the question of the active circulation of body fluids in the dentine, and the physiology of the dental tissues, an investigation which was supported by a grant of £100 from the newly established Dental Board.

Chapter 4

THE SEVENOAKS PRACTICE

At the same time as he was involved in this new investigation, Fish was hard at work building a thriving practice. His appointment diaries for 1925 show that "on a typical day he saw thirty-five patients; twenty-five, it seems, was regarded as very slack. According to a friend he expected to complete at least two fillings for each patient, with perhaps three or four gas extraction cases, and maybe a visit to the local hospital included." Saturday mornings were also reported to be very busy when about fifteen patients were seen plus one or two gas cases pushed in. In those days the family doctor gave the anaesthetic, nitrous oxide and oxygen with perhaps ethyl chloride sprayed onto a cotton mask.

The above account of his working day rather stretches the imagination when one considers the capacity of the dental engines of the time, rotating at about 3,000 revolutions a minute.

However, whatever the volume of work might have been, and it was undoubtedly large, the practice cash-book for March 1920-March 1921 shows a turnover of £4,177-10s-6d, and by 1929-30 this had reached over £9,000. If one assumes that these figures indicate Fish's own earnings for these years as being roughly £2,000 and £4,000 respectively, by today's standards this represents the equivalent of a quarter to half a million pounds per year. In the previous year, Winston Churchill as Chancellor of the Exchequer, not one of his most glorious Ministries, had reduced income tax to 4 shillings in the pound.

Despite his considerable success in Sevenoaks, Fish had his eye on higher realms, and in 1924 he obtained rooms in Cavendish Square at the bottom of Harley Street, the Mecca of doctors and dentists. In the time of Elizabeth 1st. this area had been known as Harley Fields, the property of Edward Harley, Second Earl of Oxford, and what was to become Cavendish Square was the site of the gallows, with its swinging tenant a deterrent to would-be felons. In the 18th. century the aristocracy

and persons of fashion migrated from the City of London west to the district of Marylebone. James Boswell was an early resident; Lady Nelson, the family of the Duke of Wellington, and the artist William Turner, were amongst the many peers and ambassadors that graced the area, and with them came the fashionable doctors. Gradually the number of doctors increased, for convenience to be near the hospitals and scientific institutions, and for social and professional intercourse, as well as for prestige. And of course some streets became more desirable than others, especially the southern end of Harley Street. Apparently when, in 1886, the famous doctor, Sir John Tweedy, moved northward from No.24 to No. 100 Harley Street, his older colleagues warned him that he was committing professional suicide.

Cavendish Square was without doubt the place for Fish to practise, and for the next fifteen years his time was split between his two practices and his continuing research, first at University College London and then at the Royal Dental Hospital in Leicester Square where his duties were numerous. He also found time to take part in dental politics.

After a few years of practising at Buckhurst Lodge, Fish decided that he wanted custom-built dental premises. On 15th. August 1928 he purchased a plot of land at 6 Dartford Road and had the respected London architects, Baillie Scott and Beresford, draw up plans for a single-storey building. Prior to building he grazed his horse on the land which was not far from his home. The Baillie Scott building, apart from some extension, stands today almost exactly as it was originally designed. Fish knew precisely what he wanted; three surgeries, a sterilisation room, a technician's lab with separate plaster room, office, waiting room, lavatory and garage. A unique feature was a glass dome over the entrance hall. It was here in the entrance hall that patients were greeted by the male receptionist dressed in full butler's outfit to be served with sherry while they waited; a civilised form of pre-medication still offered by the more sophisticated West End practitioner. The same attendant arrived at the beginning of the day to attend to the horses now stabled and exercised in a paddock behind the building. The surgery premises were

approached from the Dartford Road by a terrace with flower plots and massive Grecian urns, and the two rear surgeries of which Fish used one, looked out onto well tended gardens with a central fountain and trees beyond. It was a place where his well-to-do clientele including assorted celebrities could feel at home. As a colleague said, "A place of relaxation rather than fear, and with the utmost kindness Wilf encouraged his juniors in this doctrine." His standards were high and he demanded and received the best that his staff could achieve. The cast gold dentures made in later years by his technician, Derek Cudlipp, at Fish's London practice in Cavendish Square and then in Weymouth Street, are testimony to those outstanding standards.

Fish was always concerned about the public perception of his profession, and regularly propounded his belief that the status of dentistry must be founded on work of high quality. He was particularly concerned about the 1921 registered dentists, and in 1923 published letters of protest in the British Dental Journal after there was a proposal from Liverpool Dental School that they design an attenuated LDS course "for the benefit of those who have recently been admitted to the Dental Register."

Fish wrote," it is generally acknowledged that the period of four years for the diploma is none too long, and one cannot but view with dismay the proposal to grant the diploma after so short a course, however intensive it may be." And later, " lowering our standard of professional education, a result we should all deplore."

In May he wrote from Buckhurst Lodge:
"Surely if any educational body is desirous of helping these men to serve the community, the important thing is to educate them, not to provide them with an easy diploma and so confuse them utterly with the properly qualified dental surgeon.

"It is useless having an act preventing unauthorized dental practise, if, in the process of time, the standard of the authorizing diploma becomes lowered until it ceases to be any guarantee of efficiency."

On June 7th. he followed this up with a stronger letter about the educational standard of applicants for registration:

" .. concesssions both as regard the Preliminary examination, general education and the course in dental mechanics, appear to be directly conducive to the lowering of standards of professional education, a result we should all deplore..... entrants to our profession have allowed a state of intellectual discipline that will enable them to profit by the new matter that is to be laid before them in their professional studies." He was anxious to start professional training early, and goes on to suggest that "if a man has attained the age of twenty-five he will have lost much of the receptive power of the child's mind". He insisted that entrants for registration must have evidence of at least four years of approved instruction in dental mechanics, "not at the hands of unqualified operators."

These letters published in the British Dental Journal brought him to the attention of the general profession, and in a way initiated his entry into dental politics.

The Sevenoaks practice grew and assistants were taken in. In 1932 Wallace Stewart (Mac) Ross obtained part of the lease and became a partner, to be followed in 1933 by Robert Eustace, and in 1947 by Beric Southwell. They went on to expand the practice as 'Eustace and Partners' which with seven surgeries, continues to prosper to this day.

Fish was an extremely kind and generous employer, who always paid above the standard rate. When his cleaner at his house and practice at 34 Weymouth Street, where he took a lease in 1945, said that she was hard pressed to pay her bills, Fish immediately raised her wage by fifty percent. It seems that his door (or doors as he moved so frequently), was always open to his friends and junior colleagues, who received an open invitation to Sunday lunch.

Yet despite this kindness and generosity many colleagues found him aloof, and as H.M.Pickard, later professor at the Royal Dental Hospital, but then a junior colleague and friend remarked, "he was difficult to know." Others found him difficult to get close to, and many of his peers, possibly through envy, thought him too-clever-by half. As many episodes indicate he did not suffer fools gladly, especially assistants who did not come up to his

standards. At times relations with his colleagues did not run smoothly. Some photographs portray an austere face, and Lady Fish ascribed his "patrician" features to his mother, but his mischievous sense of humour to his half Irish father.

Robert Lindsay, the first full-time secretary of the BDA sent in 1926 a letter to his wife Lilian while he was attending dental conferences in the USA. He wrote that at the 7th. International Dental Congress in Philadelphia , "Fish read his paper (on the circulation of lymph in dentine and enamel) on Tuesday; I think he had a small audience. He is rather a conceited young man."

Lindsay was also critical of the quality of Fish's work, and in his diary recalls, "I saw him remove a difficult impacted molar tooth in 1929 under GA at the annual meeting of the BDA in Birmingham …. when he inadvertently removed a very large piece of the inner side of the ascending ramus of the mandible , due I am sorry to say , to a lack of concentration. At the same meeting I saw him perform an apicectomy in what I can only describe as an inexpert manner. In my small experience therefore he was not a good operator."

Lindsay goes on to comment on what he saw as bad manners in Fish's criticism of colleagues at meetings. But Fish was more satirical than bad mannered. The dental historian, Ronald Cohen, described a memorable occasion at the 1933 Annual General Meeting of the BDA in Leicester, when F.W.Broderick presented a bewildering theory of the causation of dental caries, which somehow involved the autonomic nervous system. H.R.F. Brooks, then editor of the BDJ, responded in a state of considerable excitement, "Nothing will ever convince me that there is anything of value in these papers," and refused to publish any of Broderick's submissions. Fish simply commented that the speaker, " had apparently discovered a new nervous system."

However Lindsay did conclude, "Of his out standing scientific work I am not competent to speak but he had the rare ability of being able to express himself in the spoken and written word with fluency and grace as shown by his printed speeches and several obituaries. It appears likely that he was a somewhat difficult colleague but his services to the profession are immense.

A great man."

By the time Fish left Sevenoaks in 1939 his single-minded dedication and apparently boundless energy had assured his status both professionally and financially. An item in the Evening Standard of 19th. November 1936 on Doctors' Incomes, reported that Lord Horder was earning over £20,00 per year, and Lord Dawson of Penn, the king's physician, £15,000, while the dental surgeon, Mr. Fish, " a steady £7,000-£8,000.... Mr.Fish is only forty-two ".

If one assumes that a decent annual wage at that time was £250, in today's figures these earnings are enormous, Fish's yearly income being equivalent to well over half a million pounds. In 1914 judges were paid £5,000 per year, and on this could then live in some opulence, but this salary remained the same until 1939 when it was worth a great deal less. By contrast Fish prospered through these years, and on his earnings was able to live in some style. He ran a Daimler which he called 'George', and sent his children to expensive private schools. There is a telling letter of 31st. October, 1933 from Professor F.C. Wilkinson, then Director of the Dental Hospital in Manchester, when referring a patient who worked in cancer research, " He is a very interesting fellow, but as you know, research workers are not plutocrats so deal gently with him as regards fees."

Despite Fish's considerable earnings, it seems he was 'not good with money'. He left the management of his practice completely to his secretary. She paid his earnings into the bank, and paid out all salaries and expenses. Perhaps compensating for his relatively Spartan Wesleyan upbringing , Fish enjoyed the fruits of his labours to the full. He made no investments, but bought pictures and domestic ornaments as he desired. He went to the theatre regularly, and also joined a dance club. One year, later in life, he and Lady Fish went to the Chelsea Arts Ball and took as their guests, Sir and Lady Alexander Fleming, whom he knew and worked with at St. Mary's Hospital. Despite his apparent day-to-day disinterest in money, he did make a shrewd move by not selling the Dartford Road premises to Messrs. Ross, Eustace and Southwell until 1949. During the war these two, the youngest of Fish's associates, were away in the services, and during the blitz Fish stayed with Ross in South Park, Sevenoaks.

Wallace Stewart Ross, a decade younger than Fish, was his closest friend and colleague, the man with whom at the end of a working day in Cavendish Square, over a glass or two of sherry, he would discuss all aspects of their work. Ross assisted Fish in the Hampton Hale laboratory at the Royal Dental Hospital, where together they were carrying out animal experiments on bone infection. Their conversation ranged from the design of dentures to the role of osteoclasts in bone pathology.

Ross also joined Fish in his regular deer stalking holidays in southern Ireland. One of Fish's patients was Lord Kenmare, who owned vast areas of mountain terrain around Lake Killarney, stacked with large herds of deer which destroyed the grasslands meant for sheep. Culling was necessary. Fish and Ross would shoot teal over the lake, but Fish's favourite activity lay in playing the detective game of tracking and then shooting the deer. Stalking is done in pairs, who must quietly and with considerable skill and a fund of patience, find and follow the deer until they find them in their rifle sights. Fish and Ross must have been a formidable team. According to Lady Fish, her husband was a crack shot with an excellent telescopic rifle, and aiming at a particular spot behind the head could kill a deer a mile away. Testimony to his skill was displayed by the number of massive heads that hung from the walls of Fish's homes in Esher and Storrington, a sure sign of affluence and professional success.

The deer, dripping blood, were brought down from the mountainside in the open boot of Fish's Daimler to the boos and raised fists of disapproving ramblers . Lady Fish, his second wife, was a professional painter, and while Fish indulged in blood sports in the mountains, she stayed behind to be at her easel.

Ross's son, Graeme, remembers as a boy going with these shooting parties prior to Fish's second marriage, accompanied by Maggie, for many years Fish's secretary and girl-friend, a tall, plain and rather masculine lady, whose exact relationship to Fish was uncertain. She ran the practice, and as Fish had no interest in these mundane matters, dealt with all his financial affairs.

According to Lady Fish her husband was not good with money, but as soon as Hazel married Fish she insisted that Maggie must go. When Fish died he left Maggie one of his cars, but not the Daimler.

During his first marriage Fish's home life, that is what he had of one, was not happy; the failed marriage to Hilda was the price to pay for all this success. As can happen in very early marriages, the partners mature in very different and separate ways. Apart from horse-riding and deer stalking, work had taken over Fish's life, and that was a life in which Hilda, who according to friends was a rather dull lady, could play little part, except perhaps for helping to design the gardens at their many homes. It seems that she was not his equal intellectually, and once they were old enough the two children were sent to boarding schools, James to Eton, and Vivien to Roedean, the exclusive girl's school overlooking the sea outside Brighton. Fish's relationship with his daughter must have been the most rewarding part of his home life. Vivien shared his opinions and his mischievous sense of humour, and it must have been a considerable wrench for him when in 1944 she married Neville Greaves, who worked in the shipping business. The newlyweds went to live in the Gulf where the Anglo-Iranian Oil Company attracted many Britons to that area until political turmoil drove them to more stable parts of the world. In 1951 Vivien and her husband moved to Christchurch in New Zealand, where they were to become friends of David Poswillo, an oral surgeon who was to achieve great distinction in Britain, and to become a colleague and friend of Vivien's father.

While Fish got on well with his daughter, his son James, proved to be a problem for his father. The boy, who wanted to be an actor, did badly at Eton, and when Fish was treating the Canadian tycoon, newspaper magnate and former Conservative MP, Max Aitken (made Lord Beaverbrook in 1917) he spoke about his concern for his son. Beaverbrook said that there were opportunities for young men in the prospering South African companies, and James was duly shipped off. A post with the East Geduld Mine was organised for him but lacking any training in mining he never achieved more than working in the office. In

1945 before James left England he went through the process of adopting his third Christian name, Russell (his mother's maiden name), as his surname. James claimed that this was at his father's insistence, but Fish in telling his colleague Cohen about this, said that it was James' decision. Given the ill-feeling between a disappointed father and an angry son it is possible that each saw this sorry situation in different ways, both seeing a rejection of the other's values and aspirations. Alas, James' career was not a great success, but he did made his mark in his new country in both amateur dramatics and some professional theatre. He married and had a daughter, Patricia (Trich), to whom Fish became devoted. But James' first marriage also failed; he remarried, and like his mother he died an alcoholic.

Fish had many celebrity patients including Brendan Bracken, Churchill's devoted Parliamentary Private Secretary, to whom Churchill delegated much prime ministerial authority over domestic affairs when in 1940 Churchill became Prime Minister, and prior to Clement Attlee, Leader of the Labour Party, taking over as Deputy Prime Minister. Bracken was an energetic red-haired Irishman, a very successful publisher who campaigned for Churchill when the latter stood unsuccessfully for the Leicester seat in 1923. Bracken himself was to be elected as Conservative MP for North Paddington in 1929, and became Minister of Information in Churchill's war cabinet.

But Fish's most celebrated patient was Winston Churchill himself. There is no record of exactly when Churchill became a patient, but one story proves that it was in Sevenoaks. It seems that without his partial upper denture, Churchill's speech was impaired, and when he broke the denture on a Friday and had to make a speech in the House on the following Monday, "Mr. Fish, his Sevenoaks dentist", had to be called on urgently to effect a repair. Churchill's biographer, Martin Gilbert, records letters from Churchill asking for advice on his dental problems. The first, dated 7 October 1936 reads:

"Dear Dr. Fish, The back tooth cannot be cleaned properly by a toothbrush. Will you send me a dental syringe with a right angle bend in it, so that I can wash the cavity out when I am brushing my teeth."

On 10 October Churchill wrote again to Fish: "I did not know that there was only a dressing in one of those upper teeth. Certainly the teeth are still sensitive to heat and cold. I will propose myself to see you as soon as I come again to London."

Churchill had been excluded from office since 1929. Both Prime Ministers, Ramsay MacDonald and Stanley Baldwin did not trust 'clever men' like Churchill, Beaverbrook, and the celebrated lawyer, Lord Birkenhead. Baldwin did appoint Churchill to a secret committee on research into air defence, but when Mussolini invaded Ethiopia, Churchill failed to stimulate Baldwin to any action. Baldwin's antagonism to Churchill was further heightened when in the abdication crisis in 1936 Churchill opposed Baldwin and took the side of the King.

Despite his heavy commitments Churchill came regularly to see Fish, who was at this time very involved with his work on periodontal disease, and one can imagine that he had spent much time instructing Churchill on a sound oral hygiene regime. Even during the war when he was Prime Minister Churchill carried on seeing Fish, and often took his daughter Mary with him. These appointments for treating Mary cost her father Two Guineas. Fish was always concerned about Churchill's well-being, and made sure that when Churchill was descending the stairs after leaving Fish's surgery, one nurse went ahead and one followed the great man.

In 1941, immediately before Churchill had to meet Roosevelt for the mid-Atlantic conference, Churchill developed an acute abscess on his right upper canine. Fish told him that root canal treatment was necessary, which meant that he would need to see Churchill for the next few days. Churchill insisted that this was impossible, and that Fish must sort it out right away. Ever resourceful, Fish heated a needle red hot with which he cauterised the root canal and established drainage. This emergency measure seems to have worked at least for the time being, for Churchill met Roosevelt to sign the crucial Atlantic Charter which established common principles by which Britain and the USA pursued the war.

Subsequently the tooth had to be extracted and added to the denture which is now housed, a beautiful example of cast gold work, in the museum of the Royal College of Surgeons. Encouraged by this at least temporary success, Fish used the red hot needle technique in similar situations when required, presumably under local anaesthesia.

By the end of the Second World War Fish was formally separated, although not yet divorced from his first wife. Hilda had faded from Fish's busy life and had become an alcoholic. For many years Fish maintained her in a home, and they were finally to be divorced some time before Fish was knighted. Apparently Churchill offered him a knighthood earlier, but although the stigma of divorce was not as great as it had been, Fish asked that it be delayed until the divorce was finalised. Hilda shared the burden of the road to success, but was not to know the fruits of his arrival. As soon as the divorce came through Fish re-married. His bride was Myfanwy Hazel Bruce (the Bruce referred to Scottish ancestry), the daughter of Rankin Dunlop, Senior Resident in North Borneo where she was born, and the widow of the well respected painter Francis Hodge who had been almost thirty years her senior. Hazel was eighteen years younger than Fish, and a complete contrast to Hilda Gertrude. Hazel was more attractive, better dressed and from a higher social class. She was an accomplished professional painter, having been at the Slade as a student of two famous painters, Tonks and Orpen, just following the time of Augustus John. As an honorary member of the Chelsea Arts Club Fish had met Hazel with Francis Hodge many times. Much livelier than Fish's first wife, Hazel's interests were, apart from painting especially in water colours, dancing and playing tennis; not unusual for a girl of her class. Pretty and petite, and smaller than Fish who was not a tall man, she was the perfect partner for a highly successful professional man, who by 1950 moved in elevated company. Photographs of them at meetings with other distinguished guests show Fish's evident pleasure and pride in his young wife.

Chapter 5

THE ROYAL DENTAL HOSPITAL

The centre of London from which all distances are measured is the equestrian statue of Charles I, which stands on the south side of the great open space of Trafalgar Square. A few yards to the north is Leicester Square, now a piazza, and with Piccadilly Circus to the east, the centre of London's entertainment world.

Near the south-east corner of Leicester Square is a five-story red-brick late Victorian building, the home of the Hampshire Hotel. Discrete double doors open into a smart low-ceilinged lobby, carpeted, walls of walnut veneer, and pseudo-marble faced columns divide the space. With its modern crystal chandeliers, potted plants and oil painting reproductions, it provides an atmosphere of welcome and comfort.

On a pillar by the reception desk, and no doubt overlooked by most guests, is a small brass plaque (paid for, incidentally, by the Old Students' Society) which announces:

THE
HAMPSHIRE HOTEL
occupies the building which from
1901 - 1985 housed the
ROYAL DENTAL HOSPITAL
and
SCHOOL OF DENTAL SURGERY
the oldest dental school in the United Kingdom.
These institutions opened in Soho in 1858 and
1859 and later moved to this site.

Gone is the old tiled floor lobby with its iron-gated lift that took apprehensive patients and busy staff to all treatment floors; gone the stairs down to the staff and student cloakrooms and store rooms where white coats were handed out; gone the watchful Jack Knights, porter and head porter from 1924 for the next forty years.

Although it was not the first dental hospital (it was beaten by a few months by the Birmingham and Midland Dental Dispensary), as the Dental Hospital of London it was the first dental teaching institution in England. It was the offspring of the Odontological Society of London, a society largely dominated by the Memorialists, and as such it came within the orbit of the Royal College of Surgeons of England.

Its formation did not go uncontested. The Independents, a group of dentists that disliked the dominance of the Royal College (RCS), fought hard to set up their own College of Dentists, but without success.

When looking at the state of organisation of dentistry and training for the profession at that time, it has to be kept in mind that in 1858 only one third of those engaged in the practice of medicine possessed a formal qualification. The regulation of dentistry was part of the movement to regulate the medical professions. There was no defined curriculum of training or formal qualification, and the RCS was well placed to organise these matters. Dentistry as a profession in Britain is very much the child of the Royal College of Surgeons, and the history of dentistry as a profession in Britain is marked by its preoccupation with its relationship to medicine. Although British dentistry throughout the twentieth century became increasingly independent of medicine, it does not possess the autonomy that the American profession so values. Fish would never have countenanced autonomy; he was always insistent on dentistry being a branch of medicine. The essential problem was how to synthesise the 'art' of dentistry within the science of medical knowledge, a subject dear to Fish's philosophy.

In the infancy of the profession the establishment of a dental school gave it some independence from medicine. As Smith and Cottell write in their history of the RDH, the dentists became masters in their own house, encouraged to develop the profession in a way they wanted. Unfortunately independence from the governance of any general hospital or medical school proved in the long run to have disadvantages which unravelled over the years, and in the end resulted in the closure of the RDH in 1985.

The other dental schools developed within the umbrella of a medical institution, either school or hospital. Usually this development had the support of the parent institution, but this was not so in the case of Guy's.

After gaining his medical and dental diplomas, F. Newland Pedley, son of a dentist in Australia, went to Guy's Hospital, becoming Dental Surgeon in 1887. His clinic amounted to one room with two dental chairs, which he ran largely at his own expense. With the increasing demand for treatment it became obvious that more help, in particular in the form of students was needed. But Pedley's ideas for a dental school met with opposition from the Guy's establishment. Undeterred Pedley encouraged his staff to send patients to Leicester Square where the Royal Dental Hospital already had enough patients to cope with. As Pedley said, "we filled their staircases" to the point where the RDH had to complain to Guy's, who only then saw the light. Pedley also played a part in the formation of the Royal Army Dental Corps, once again against the opposition of the medical establishment. He volunteered to serve in the Boer War and promoted the idea of a formal unit to serve the dental needs of the soldiers; the Great War saw this established.

The foundation of the London Hospital Dental School highlights the differences between the establishment of the various schools. Its terms of reference conformed to the recommendations of the new Dental Council. The Royal Commission of 1910 was set up to examine education in London with special reference to the organisation of London University. This asked for a submission from the Dental Council, and the Council's reply has been summarised as follows:

1. Dentistry is a branch of medicine because of the relationship between general and dental disease, and the dentist needs knowledge of such related diseases. This view is emphasised because "owing to the elaboration of the art, the science of the dental surgeon is in danger of being eclipsed ". As a consequence, general subjects such as Chemistry, Anatomy, Physiology, etc., are important to the dental surgeon, and

medical and dental education should be along "identical or parallel lines".

2. The diploma is adequate as a qualification to practise but a degree would permit a wider education and attract those of higher ability, would stimulate research and the perfection of technique.

3. Apprenticeship is fatally marred by the need of the practitioner to delegate instruction of the apprentice to the mechanics.

4. Dental education is obviously best carried out in a well equipped dental school which is part of a "General Medical School".

5. Supervision of the courses should be carried out by a dental board on which elected representatives of the dental schools would sit.

Two other factors were regarded as of considerable importance. The first was the standard of the teaching staff, a concern of the Governors of Guy's Hospital, manifesting that proud loyalty that marks the Guy's man, when they insisted that the staff of the dental school must be worthy of Guy's Hospital. The RDH had no such external supervisory body. The second was the financial resources of the institution. Fish's time at the RDH was dogged by limitations in both these areas.

The Medical Committee of the RDH was fundamentally conservative. Any change in the essential organisation of the institution was usually resisted, and in the beginning the views of the Medical Committee, i.e. the part-time 'Honoraries', or 'consultants' as they would be called today, decided on the direction of the school. This continued until Professor Harry Stobie was appointed as the first full-time Dean, a position he held from 1920 to 1948.

Prior to 1910 payment to part-time clinical staff was "largely hypothetical", and even after the University Grants Committee gave grants for education, mainly for clinical teaching, these "consultants" received very little remuneration. As late as 1970 this amounted to £50 per year for each half day of teaching per week.

However by providing their services these men (for the

professional staff were all male) were not only fulfilling a public duty, but adding prestige to their practices and gaining access to hospital facilities for their oral surgery. The Royal Dental Hospital was closely connected to Charing Cross Hospital which was then scarcely two hundred yards away across the Charing Cross Road. Many men were honorary members of the staff of both establishments, and Harley Street was under a mile away. Such a comfortable combination of advantages was difficult to disturb.

At the establishment of the school its legal obligation had been "to provide the Poorer Classes with Gratuitous Advice and Surgical Aid in Diseases and Irregularities of the teeth". But in 1924 a year before Fish was appointed to the school, this version had been changed "to provide advice and treatment for poor persons in connection with their teeth." In a word, patients receiving treatment could be charged. Fees were already charged for dentures and this arrangement was extended to all operative procedures, and in 1928 an almoner was appointed to assess the fees. As a consequence of patient payments the financial situation was made more secure.

The budgetary condition of the hospital had always been precarious. A good example of this problem related to the acceptance of women students. In 1912 Douglas Gabell, an Honorary Dental Surgeon and lecturer in Prosthetics, who was to become a guide and friend to Fish, proposed to the Medical Committee ,"That ladies be eligible as students and pupils at the Royal Dental Hospital of London", but this difficult decision was postponed. However with the outbreak of war the number of men entering the school was dramatically reduced, and total fees received dropped from £3,452 in 1913/14 to £898 in 1915/16. Inevitably it followed that women were accepted, and of the twenty-five students accepted in 1916-18, ten were women.

But the hospital was still pressed for money, and when in 1918 the committee planned to purchase the neighbouring piece of land on Orange Street to provide room to extend the hospital for in-patient facilities, the Dean, W.H.Dolamore, advertised in The Westminster Gazette for what today we would call a "white knight" to come to the rescue. The fact that the RDH was independent of both a medical school and a hospital meant that it had somehow to fend for itself, and at times of financial crisis a connection with a medical school was frequently discussed.

The institution did have a symbolic white knight for in 1919 The Prince of Wales had agreed to become President of the Royal Dental Hospital of London in recognition of the institution's services. The reputation of the dental hospital was further enhanced when Sir Frank Colyer, then in the chair, agreed to a suggestion from the Medical Officer of the Borough of Ealing that the already established scheme for the treatment of children at the hospital be continued.

Former staff had returned from the War, patient attendance was rising sharply, and the establishment to which Fish was to become attached was a thriving and respected dental institution. In 1921 the Chancellor of the Exchequer allowed an increase of £500,000 to universities and colleges, and the University Grants Committee allowed RDH a grant of £500 for 1921-22. Also in that year the Medical Committee after much resistance resolved, "That it is desirable that the degree of Bachelor of Dental Surgery be instituted for Internal and External students." No doubt this forward looking move was made under pressure from the University Grants Committee, but it did not seem to affect the basically conservative attitude of the "honoraries". When Douglas Gabell, now chairman of the Medical Committee, reported that the school could get all the photographic equipment it wanted , including a half-plate camera, lens and accessories, for £50, the idea was not taken up. The Honorary Dental Surgeons were not ready for such innovation. Even in 1936 when Fish proposed hiring a cinematic projector to help with lectures, the Board of Management decided to " leave the matter on the table." By then Fish had used photography to good effect for his own research and as illustrations for his books.

The volume of clinical work at the hospital grew, and its function as a dental dispensary was greatly appreciated. Goodwill to the hospital was demonstrated when the RDH Dramatic Society was formed, and at its first performance on 5th.

October 1924 at the Alhambra Theatre in Leicester Square, some of the most famous performers of the day, Gracie Fields, Jack Buchanan, Will Fyfe, Stanley Holloway and George Robey, all gave their services free.

Such help was badly needed because after the immediate post-war intake of student numbers of around 100, by 1928 that had sunk to 20, and in the 'thirties the average annual entry was 27. Patient waiting lists were in the hundreds, and the demand for prosthetics was so great that a full-time technician had to be taken on. Unpaid 'clinical assistants' were sought after, and moves to amalgamate with a medical school not already connected with a dental institution, were broached but to no avail.

By this time power had drifted from the Medical Committee to the Board of Management which constitutionally had always had ultimate authority. On occasion these two bodies did not see eye to eye, and Fish's relationship with the institution that finally led to his resignation was affected by this conflict.

The relationship of these two bodies was further complicated by the hospital's connection with London University. In 1918 Stobie had been appointed full-time professor in Dental Surgery, and in 1920 the University of London introduced its dental degree, the BDS. Initially, as stated, the school was very reluctant to accept it. The continuing argument about the relationship of dentistry to medicine raised its head, now compounded by the relationship between the Royal Colleges and the university. With only a diploma of the Royal Colleges as the formal dental qualification, dentistry was firmly within the dominion of medicine, but as a university discipline that dominance was challenged.

A further difficulty with the degree was that entry to the BDS course demanded matriculation, while the LDS RCS course only required the College of Preceptors certificate or its equivalent, a less onerous demand. The prejudice against the BDS course was so strong that the Dental Board would only give grants to needy students taking the LDS, and even in 1947 only 2 out of 86 students were taking the degree. In the other schools, especially in the provinces, the degree was much more readily accepted.

Also universities demanded full-time academic commitment and an element of research. When Stobie was appointed he had to relinquish all private practice, and many young potential teachers, who started as part-time demonstrators or researchers, drifted off into lucrative private practice. W. Stewart Ross, who worked as a research assistant with Fish for many years in the Hale Laboratory, and became one of Fish's partners in the Sevenoaks practice as well as in Cavendish Square, was one of these. When working on a monkey in experiments to study the metabolism of dental tissues, MacRoss, as everyone called him, demonstrated that irritation to the dental pulp could stimulate the deposition of secondary cementum.

As a very busy dental dispensary and training institution, clinical work and teaching filled the day and little time was left for research activity, which in any case, had been suspended since 1914. In 1912 at the suggestion of two eminent staff members, J.G.Turner and W.Warwick James, the Medical Committee had reluctantly agreed that some of the facilities could be used for research, but only in the evening and on subjects that had its approval. Also any publication had to acknowledge the debt to the Committee.

William Warwick James OBE, MCh, FRCS, has been described as one of the most memorable dentists of his generation, and demonstrated the versatility common in many professional careers before the days of specialisation. After serving a dental apprenticeship, he took an LDS at the RDH, medicine at the Middlesex Hospital and obtained an FRCS in 1905. As a student he had heard the last course of lectures on dental anatomy given by Charles Tomes. Apart from his dental activities, he was a shrewd business man, and in 1905 bought the long leases on what was to become prime property close to Regent's Park, numbers 2 and 3 Park Crescent for a modest sum. At that time the smoke from the steam trains in nearby Great Portland Street made these properties almost uninhabitable, but Warwick James foresaw that the lines would within two years be electrified. He converted the houses to provide many dental surgeries which were still being used fifty years later. In his free time he played the 'cello with professional musicians, and according to his obituary, he was a friend of T.E.Lawrence (of Arabia) and his mother.

In 1914, Warwick James, with RDH colleagues Gabell and Payne, published a book on Odontomes. During the war he was called upon to treat jaw injuries, and received an OBE for his services. Many years later, at the beginning of the Second World War, Warwick James and Ben Fickling, who had also obtained his FRCS, produced a book on 'Injuries to the Jaws and Face'.

In 1913 Mrs. John Hale, widow of John Hampton Hale, a former chairman of the Management Committee, gave One Thousand Pounds for research equipment for studies on a broad range of subjects, but giving priority to Bacteriology and Clinical Pathology. Even then facilities were minimal and prior to the war little research was carried out. The provision of treatment was the hospital's primary obligation. But in 1926 the new and forward looking Dental Board of the United Kingdom provided a grant of £1,000 for structural work and equipment to the John Hampton Hale Research Laboratory.

On July 16th. 1925, with Turner's backing, Fish was appointed Honorary Assistant Dental Surgeon for a period of five years, when his post would be eligible for renewal. He came with references from Colyer, and from his Dean at the Manchester Medical School, Professor John S. B. Stopford, who described Fish's research for his MD thesis as a first rate piece of work

Although individuals might have a particular interest in a dental speciality, such as prosthetics or orthodontics, staff members' duties were wide ranging, and Fish's duties included teaching prosthetics as well as all those other tasks that fell to the "Honorary" to perform, including oral surgery and restorative dentistry. Fish was also keen to pursue the research he had already started at UCL.

J.G.Turner FRCS, whose father had been a founder of the BDA, was the first director of the Hale Laboratory, the foundation of which, according to Fish's obituary of Turner, was the fulfilment of a long-held dream. Although a clinician, Turner had started the practice of having routine clinical material sectioned for histological examination. Fish describes him as a link, along with Howard Mummery, to the scientific pioneers, John and Charles Tomes. Turner had been on the staff of the RDH since 1895, and therefore when Fish was appointed to the staff, Turner was a very senior Honorary Dental Surgeon, even senior to Warwick James. He had published works on dental anatomy and oral pathology, as well as on the relationship between diet and dental caries, and his appointment to the directorship of the laboratory is not surprising.

In 1925 the Dental Board had provided Fish with a grant for £100 for one year, and it seems doubtful whether the reinstatement of the Hampton Hale Laboratory would have got off to such a good start without Fish's energy and research experience at University College. His reputation as a research worker was established and his grant was renewed the following year.

Up to that time whatever research work carried out at the RDH tended to be of an institutional nature and decided by committee. Fish was a free spirit and not likely to be subject to the decision of a body of clinicians or laymen, some of whom he could not regard with respect. His work at UCL on the lymph supply of the dental tissues had been well received by the Odontological Section of the Royal Society of Medicine, of which Douglas Gabell was then president, and he had the Dental Board of the United Kingdom behind him. He had begun to establish an international reputation when he lectured on 'The Circulation of Lymph in Dentine and Enamel' at The Seventh International Dental Congress held in Philadelphia in 1926. His detractors were powerless to frustrate his research programme; nevertheless one decade later they did just that.

At the time Fish joined the RDH, unlike the situation in American schools, little advanced conservative work was carried out. Colyer's obsession with focal infection meant that the main clinical activities centred on extractions and the provision of dentures. An important move was made around 1930 when several young demonstrators were sent to American schools for a few months to learn advanced operative techniques. When they came back they completely revolutionised the teaching of conservative dentistry at the RDH, and, as Fish reports, the movement rapidly spread to all the other English schools.

Chapter 6

PROSTHETICS

As a senior member of the RDH staff and a respected teacher of prosthetics, and then as a friend, Douglas Gabell played an important role in the early stage of Fish's career. Like many prominent teachers of his generation Gabell started his career articled as a dental mechanic in Brighton, before entering the Dental Hospital of London (renamed RDH) and qualifying in dentistry, and subsequently in medicine at Charing Cross Hospital Medical School. As an Honorary Dental Surgeon Gabell was also a lecturer in dental mechanics. He wrote a popular teaching text, "Dental Prosthetics" and became an examiner to the young Dental Board of the United Kingdom.

In the same year that Fish joined the staff of the RDH Gabell retired due to ill-health, and when he died soon after, Fish lost one of his best friends and supporters.

When Fish took over the lectureship in prosthetics, dentures were made from cast gold or vulcanite, the product of hardened rubber and a bye-product of the new motor car tyre industry. Plaster of Paris or 'composition' were used as impression materials, each with its devotees for specific use. Where the alveolar anatomy involved no or very minor undercuts, plaster was the obvious choice, but where maxillary tuberosities and other convexities were present the more flexible composition material was required. Special trays provided more even pressure over uneven ridges, and Fish made these as a matter of course. As he explained many years later, his research into denture design was provoked by the demand for dentures at a time, especially in the 'twenties, when doctors advised the wholesale extraction of teeth suspected of being the source of focal infection.

In the early 'thirties the first hydrocolloids made their appearance, only gradually to replace plaster of Paris, and acrylic resins were at an experimental stage. Advances in these new materials were made in the USA, and British dentists were very slow to take them up. Indeed, when in 1948 dentures became free of charge under the National Health Service, the demand for the replacement of ancient and broken vulcanite dentures, often, because of the cost of new ones, worn for over twenty years on diminishing alveolar ridges, was of avalanche proportions.

In making functional dentures the primary concern had always been their fit, and therefore the accurate registration of the alveolar ridges, i.e. the impression surfaces.

The importance of the biting or occlusal surfaces of dentures, in both resting and functional relationship, had been recognised as early as the eighteenth century, and Fish's teaching included descriptions of the Curves of Spee and Monson, which occur in nature, as Fish writes, "in order that during mastication as many surfaces of as many teeth as possible shall grind at the same moment." Increasingly sophisticated articulators were devised for registering functional relationships and movements. Again, these advances were made largely in the USA.

The history of prosthetic dentistry is long, and the literature on denture design and construction voluminous, yet systematic and detailed attention to the oral anatomy seems to have received less attention than might be expected. Much of the early research in Prosthetics, mainly carried out in the USA, gave most attention to dental materials and the mechanical aspects of design and construction. This may well have been a consequence of the guarded autonomy of the American dental profession and the separation of dental from medical school teaching. Research and the teaching of anatomy and physiology in US dental schools was much enhanced in the mid-thirties by the flight of Jewish research workers from Nazi persecution. This brought to dental histology, anatomy and physiology in the USA, such great names as Gottlieb, Orban, Weinmann and Sicher, and many others. Their subsequent influence in Europe was as a backwash from the opportunities offered by the American schools. Fish always acknowledged his debt to these workers, especially to Gottlieb, and correspondence between them demonstrates a high regard for each others' work.

In the introduction to the first edition of his ,"Principles of Full

Denture Prosthesis", which appeared in 1932, Fish writes, "An attempt is here made to systematise the modelling of the whole of each surface of the denture, and to base it upon an appreciation of definite physical laws, anatomical structures and physiological processes."

Fish dedicated this first edition to the memory of Douglas Phillimore Gabell, and in his introduction he writes, "… my late predecessor Mr. Douglas Gabell to whose memory this book is dedicated in token of the high esteem in which he is held by his old school and as a mark of respect for the value of his teaching on the importance of the molar flange in full lower dentures." In the same introduction Fish also thanks Professor H.A.Harris, who as a senior demonstrator in the anatomy department at University College, was Fish's advisor for his MD research and in subsequent investigations. Harris or 'H.A.' as his students called him, had an illustrious career; he was Hunterian professor at the Royal College of Surgeons, and became Professor of Anatomy at Cambridge in 1934. Fish also acknowledges his debt to Dr.(later Professor) D.T.Harris who advised on the research that Fish carried out at the physiology department of UCL from 1925-27. This was part of the experimental investigation of enamel, dentine and the dental pulp, which was to earn him a Doctor of Science degree in 1933.

A further dimension to Fish's activity had come earlier with his appointment to the staff of St. Mary's Hospital in November 1928. Earlier that year St. Mary's Medical Committee had considered applications for the posts of Dental Surgeon from several applicants, including Fish. Herbert Smale was appointed as Dental Surgeon, and Fish as a 'supernumerary' with a view to his appointment as Assistant Dental Surgeon "when the necessary alterations have been made to the Standing Rules of the Hospital, to permit of such an appointment being made." At the proposal of a Dr. Wilfred Harris, Standing Rule 78 was modified "to permit of the appointment of an Assistant Dental Surgeon as a member of the Medical Staff of the Hospital", and Fish was appointed for 5 years. He was now on the Medical Committee with Mr. Smale and a Dr. A. Fleming.

In these years he was also in practice in both Sevenoaks and in Cavendish Square.

He still lived in Sevenoaks, and must have worked out a timetable and itinerary which took in mornings at the RDH in Leicester Square for some teaching, and then research in the Hale laboratory or at UCL in Gower Street, some morning clinics at St.Mary's as well as research there, and afternoons in clinical practice at 9 Cavendish Square. He admits to spending more time in practice than in research work, and probably did all his writing at home. He put in two men's work every week.

Early on in his time in the prosthetic department at RDH, Fish wrote an article in the RDH Reports of 1926, in which he expressed the view, "It is one of the oldest fallacies of our profession, and certainly one that has led to the expenditure of more fruitless ingenuity than any other, that the stability of a denture depends upon suction." In his book Fish also expresses concern about the limitations of occlusal balance. "Unfortunately," he writes, "there has grown up a heresy that balancing the occlusion will help to stabilise a denture during mastication. It will not; it will only avoid to some extent the inevitable tendency of the occlusal surface to unstabilise the appliance. There is a fundamental difference between actively "stabilising" a denture, and merely avoiding a source of instability. In exerting a force on the food by pressing against it to crush it, an equal and opposite force is exerted on the occlusal surface by the food and some component of this force will inevitably tend to dislodge the denture."

He went on to formulate "a rule for the occlusal surface", which in his book he emphasises in italics, "The reciprocal pressure between the dentures must be concentrated in the premolar region, and must act in an upward and backward direction on the upper, and in a downward in forward direction in the lower denture." He made further detailed analysis of the forces on partial and complete dentures in function. In his book Fish pays considerable attention to the details of impression taking and to the occlusion, important points being reinforced by drawings made by Miss Eleanor Dale, and photographs by himself. A novel feature of the book was the page set-up. Only one side of the page was written on so that text and illustration can be referred to simultaneously. Another unique feature was the use of stereoscopic photography to highlight the modelling of impressions and models, so that the details of the oral anatomy are emphasised. It is in this attention to the oral soft tissues, and in particular to muscle activity that he makes his most important contribution to denture design. He called the polished surfaces of the denture, "the third surface", that is the one that fits against the moveable tissues of the cheeks, the lips and tongue. As Fish says, "these have hardly been dealt with at all," yet it is in "the modelling of these surfaces which determine the position of the arch on the ridge" and which "harnesses the very considerable muscular power of the buccinator, orbicularis orbis, tongue and other muscles."

In more detail he continues, "The polished surface of the dentures should exhibit a series of inclined planes to the muscles of the tongue and the cheeks which will cause these muscles to push the denture into place. The lingual surface of the upper looks inwards and downwards, and the lower inwards and upwards. The buccal surface of the upper (denture) looks outwards and downwards, and of the lower outwards and upwards."

"Flanges on the lower denture should extend under the buccinator muscle, and under the tongue to act as 'handles' to enable these muscles to hold the denture in place."

"The lower denture must have a narrow arch, in the premolar region to avoid being lifted by the corners of the mouth."

The anatomical descriptions in the Third Edition of his book, which appeared in 1937, were based upon recent dissections carried out in the anatomy department of Manchester University, his alma mater, and in his teaching of prosthetics he referred his students to articles in the anatomy journals.

Requests for the First Edition came from all over the world, including the USA and Australia. Reviews were immensely enthusiastic, and appeared in many of the European dental journals. The review in 'Oral Topics' declared, " Dr. Fish's work is the greatest advance that has been made in denture architecture in recent years." The BDJ was equally enthusiastic, " His policy is not a mere reiteration of the time honoured principles of muscle trimming, but ... he shows how these muscles not only can but must be brought to our aid by so shaping the polished surface that they will be enabled to hold the denture in place." And " Fish has, in his inimitable way, sent toppling many of the theories which have bound dental surgeon and his mechanic for many years. It is doubtful whether most of the dental surgeons will agree with the author's statement that full lower dentures are much easier to stabilise than full uppers, but perhaps when we have followed his advice carefully we shall change our opinion."

In 1964 the Sixth Edition, edited by Professor Ernest Matthews of Manchester, appeared at a price of 36 shillings. The review of that edition in the Journal of the Royal Society of Medicine described the book as "a classic in the literature of dental prosthetics...Nobody can study it without being more enlightened in the end and helped with the problem denture."

Fish was not a charismatic lecturer, but he was extremely articulate and highly organised, and no doubt from listening to his father's sermons, he had a considerable facility with the English language. This ability plus his clear and logical presentation of facts supported by appropriate analogies, allowed him to command his audiences, whether students or seasoned practitioners. Also he was a very experienced clinician, and recognised the problems of the ordinary dental practitioner. Even though he worked on a more elevated plane, Fish was a man with whom they could identify. He was not one of those ivory tower specialists or professors, of whom by the mid-thirties there were a growing number. Fish knew that even the most carefully designed appliance could present problems. He recognised that in some patients with extremely sensitive oral mucosa, even the most perfectly made denture might not always be comfortable, and writes," ..in some cases, after total extraction of the teeth, the soft tissues covering the mutilated lower jaw are too sensitive to bear the pressure of the most perfectly constructed denture with anything approaching comfort...but even in these patients their problem would be helped if dentures were perfectly accurately fashioned."

He recognised that he preached a counsel of perfection, and wrote at the conclusion of the introduction to his Third Edition in 1937, " Specialists in dental prosthesis will perhaps complain that the face bow and adjustable articulator are not given the place of honour they deserve, and that the plaster lower impression is a lazy escape from the tedious but valuable method of building an impression step by step in composition. They may say that the muscle trimmed upper composition impression is incomparably the best and should be used exclusively ....My apologies are due to them, but these methods are too tedious for application to appliances made by a busy man in a poor district, and too full of pitfalls for anyone who has only one or two full denture cases a year in a practice amongst people who come to him because he is expert in saving - not replacing- their teeth. The specialist himself is not in need of any instruction in these matters."

The first edition of the book was an immediate sell-out, and in April, Fish's publisher, John Bale, wrote to him, " this book has gone out of print... if you stand to make it a second edition we think that should be delayed for a couple of months before publishing."

A revised edition came out the following year, and a third edition in 1937. By this time Fish had been appointed Assistant Honorary Dental Surgeon to St. Mary's Hospital in Paddington.

Whatever the importance of Fish's research in the physiology of the dental tissues, which brought him recognition and respect amongst his fellow research workers in Britain and in other countries, his book on prosthetics further enhanced his reputation in the profession at large. He, together with his senior technician, Mr. Charles Phillimore, were in constant demand for lectures and demonstrations, and copies of his models were sought after like trophies of an ideal. Of course there were critics. A.G.Allen, who was a prosthetist at the London Hospital Dental School, was dismissive of Fish's ideas of denture design, and claimed that he had been teaching that approach for years. According to Professor Miles, who a few years later joined the staff of the

London, Allen did not want to admit that the merit of Fish's approach was not as the result of a piecemeal approach to a clinical problem, so characteristic of most work at that time, but as a system based on principles which rest on sound anatomical understanding.

Not every patient was perfectly happy with Fish's dentures, and one of these became a patient of Ronald Cohen, the respected historian of British dentistry, who when in practice saw one of Fish's patients. He wrote that " her dentures were the most beautiful I have ever seen with a great deal of gold incorporated in them and of course they were constructed according to Fish's theories." Alas the only problem was that the patient couldn't wear them either to speak or eat., and refused to return to Fish for re-examination. The most distinguished problem patient was Winston Churchill, for whom Fish made a partial upper denture. The story is one that Fish always delighted in telling against himself. Apparently, with Churchill in the chair, Fish informed him that he had written a book about dentures. Not too happy with the appliance, Churchill delayed payment, but when he did pay, the cheque came with a letter with the comment, I know you have written a book about dentures, but I think you should read one! The remark was no doubt typical of Churchill's wicked humour, and made tongue in cheek because Churchill continued to be a regular and devoted patient. Indeed the famous novelist, Compton Mackenzie is supposed to have said that the war was won on a denture. "Without the four front teeth his speech was indistinct", and if Churchill's rhetoric was a factor in the victory, the unseen hand of Fish was an important part of the war effort.

In later years Fish decided that the tongue was a major cause of denture instability, and he made plaster cast of the space required by the tongue so that the lingual aspect of the polished surface of the lower denture could be redesigned.

Fish's analytic and systematic way of thinking about problems that presented in practise, represents the essence of Fish's contribution to clinical dentistry. It was appreciated by the profession at large, but resented by some of his peers.

Even Colyer, with whom Fish had worked at Sidcup Hospital

after the Great War, was reluctant to praise Fish, although he respected his sharp brain. Respect moderated by envy of his success, and suspicion of this obviously ambitious and thrusting man, seems to have marked Fish's relations with many of his colleagues. However that did not appear to deter him. He carried on with his experimental work and histological studies of dental physiology and of caries and periodontal disease.

Chapter 7

WORK AT THE HAMPTON HALE

Once the equipment in the Hampton Hale laboratory was set up, Fish's research into the physiology of the dental tissues could be pursued in earnest. The animal house was established in semi-permanent buildings on the roof of the RDH, and like most structures of that nature, especially given the chronic financial difficulties at the RDH, they were to last for many years after Fish's time.

Fish had to start almost from scratch. As he recorded later, the laboratory in 1928 had only one slide of periodontal disease, a decalcified section, while at that time Gottlieb in Vienna had thousands of slides of a diversity of conditions.

The laboratory equipment was basic but of good quality. As Pickard comments," by today's standard it would represent a degree of poverty almost beyond belief." It had all that was thought necessary at the time for histological work on hard and soft tissues, and for research on animals as was then required. Hard sections were produced by grinding, and soft sections produced from decalcified specimens embedded in paraffin and cut on a Cambridge rocking microtome. A "sledge" microtome, celloidin embedding and frozen sections all followed in due course. The main microscope used by Fish was a binocular Leitz with a wide range of lenses, and in time a phase contrast system was added. Other members of staff used less advanced microscopes.

A Leitz monocular microscope was used for photomicrography. This was carried on a bench with a 'Ponitolite' light source, condenser lenses, and a quarter plate bellows camera which gave high quality results. There were facilities for bacteriological studies, often used by Dr. I.H. MacLean, the bacteriologist from St. Mary's Hospital.

Fish's experiments used a wide range of animals, cats, dogs, even monkeys, and a variety of rodents. The larger animals were to be a source of considerable friction with the committees, many members of which seemed to disapprove of the use of animals. Fish was to find that the general atmosphere around research at RDH was not as happy as at the physiology department at UCL. At times it is difficult to distinguish precisely where any specific piece of work was carried out, and of course, Fish carried out a fair amount of microscopic work at home, well into the small hours.

H.A. Harris, who had helped Fish with his MD research at UCL, became a close friend and frequently enjoyed the hospitality of Dr. and Mrs. Fish. Those were the days when following entertainment to lunch or dinner a formal letter of thanks arrived in the first post the next day. Harris's letters reveal a cheerful intimacy. Fish, whose favourite tipple was dry sherry, must have been a generous and jovial host. In one postcard, coming after what must have been a splendid evening of conversation of a philosophical turn, Harris writes, "This triumph for Nonconformity - religious, intellectual and social is good for us all." In those few words Harris summarised the stance that Fish took in all aspects of his work, the fruit of his Wesleyan inheritance.

Once Fish was firmly established on the hospital ladder his life became even busier.

He was an active member of the RDH Medical Committee, and an increasingly prominent member of the British Dental Association. He was seen to be at the cutting edge of dental science, and as his reputation grew he became a popular lecturer at BDA branch and district meetings up and down the country.

Prosthetics and his work on the physiology and pathology of the dental tissues were his prime interests, but harvesting funds for the Hale laboratory was always a problem. The Medical Committee appeared to be more interested in raising funds for the Athletic Club. Smith and Cottell report that when in 1923 money was needed for a sports ground of their own and the sports committee asked for help "The Medical Committee responded to this request with enthusiasm. Within a month the Dean announced that two members of the Committee of Management had offered contributions - Sir Fisher Dilkes was prepared to lend £1,000 on mortgage and Mr. H. Haynes said he would meet 10% of the purchase price. The Students' Club was able to provide £1,000 , and the Medical Committee agreed to "invest £1,600 from the funds of the school. Members of the Committee themselves contributed £600, and the thing was done."

This was in distinct contrast to the fact that Fish had to pay his personal grant money into supporting the laboratory. By this time his work on the metabolism of the dental tissues was well under way. In April 1928 he was able to report to the Medical Branch of the Board of Education that his perfusion studies had demonstrated among other findings that:

a) there is a lymph circulation in the dentinal tubules of the monkey and dog,

b) enamel prisms sheaths in the dog are irrigated with lymph almost to the surface of the enamel

c) monkey enamel is almost devoid of lymph except in the occasional lamellae

d) the continuity of the cuticle, lamellae and prism sheaths suggest that they are all of the same biochemical nature, i.e. keratinous or pre-keratinous.

Despite the progress of Fish's work, the Board of Education debated whether to continue his grant. By this time some conflict had arisen with the theories put forward by Mrs. May Mellanby, a research worker with a considerable reputation, as well as influence in both the medical and dental professions. Even more important, she was the wife of Dr. (later Sir) Edward Mellanby, a powerful member of the Medical Research Council. A critical letter from Bedford College for Women criticising Fish's work, accuses him of publishing his results and conclusions with "too little evidence", and not giving due acknowledgement to previous workers in the field. This seems to be the first sign of a feud that would continue for the next decade.

In 1929 the expenditure of the laboratory exceeded income by £468 and Fish provided for the greater part of the deficiency from his own research grant. In July of that year the minutes of the Medical Committee record a gift from Fish of a desk, chairs and an electric fire, as well as a binocular microscope. Fish could well afford such gifts. His practice in Sevenoaks with several partners was booming, and his West End practice was adorned by celebrities of whom perhaps the best known were Winston Churchill and the newspaper proprietor, Beaverbrook.

The minutes for the year 1932 show that Fish was involved in completing his research on the dental tissues at University College, as well as in a diversity of activities at the RDH.

He was on the committee that decided that in all general anaesthetic (gas) cases the throat pack had to be placed by an anaesthetist and not a student. Those were the days when complete tooth clearances were common, and students vied with each other to reach a thousand extractions. One dreads to think of the objects inhaled or swallowed that provoked that resolution. Deaths were not unknown when the depth of anaesthesia was judged by the shade of blue reached by the patient's complexion.

Firm decisions were rarely reached at Medical Committee meetings, and many matters were referred to sub-committees. Fish was appointed to the appliance sub-committee, and when a request came from the BDA for help in organising a joint meeting with the Canadian Dental Association Fish was appointed to its chair.

This sub-committee was responsible for drawing up the syllabus for teaching dental mechanics. The making of models was a routine activity and naturally Fish arranged the exhibits for the Canadian visit. At the time he was carrying out research on muscle-trimmed composition impressions, and this proved to be an opportunity for his reputation to cross the Atlantic.

He did in fact cross the Atlantic in the Duchess of York of the Canadian Pacific Steamship Line, according to its logo the "world's greatest transit system", and on board worked on the final draft of the introduction to his research report.

On 5th. August 1932 he wrote to his secretary, Miss Winifred Milward, with detailed instructions about retyping and keeping a carbon copy of all new typescript. "Keep this manuscript in the safe at night," he enjoined.

He wrote, " The experiments recorded in this report having

extended over a period of eight years, it seemed desirable to publish the findings in their present form, not because any finality had been reached, but because sufficient facts had accumulated to render possible a fairly connected account of the reaction of the dentine and dental pulp to caries and to other lesions of the dentine."

This statement and indeed the work itself is typical of his meticulous care with all aspects of the work, and his ability to express his findings with clarity and concision.

The visit to Canada, as expressed by many letters of thanks from all over the country, was a great success. Two dentists, Drs. Scott and Clarke travelled over 2,000 miles to the conference and to witness Fish's presentations. He gave a paper on his work on the lymph supply to dentine, as well as demonstrations of his prosthetic techniques which achieved extraordinary popularity. So far as the general dental practitioner was concerned this was work of everyday practical importance.

His prestige as a clinician and scientist was firmly secured across the Atlantic, as well as closer to home. A letter to Fish on 2nd. December 1933 came to 31 Queen Anne Street where he then practised, from the Irish Dental Society enclosing a cheque for the handsome sum of Ten Guineas to cover travelling expenses.

His stature was also recognised in Australia. In the autumn of 1935 Fish made the journey to Australia at the invitation of the Dental Board of Victoria in Melbourne.

The telegram of invitation informed him that all his expenses would be paid together with a fee of Five Hundred Pounds Sterling, a magnificent sum in those days.

While there he gave lectures and demonstrations of his histological research and his prosthetics, and received an Honorary D.D.S. from the university. As always his technique for designing the full lower denture attracted great attention. He received many letters of thanks and congratulations, but one of the most important events was Fish's meeting with H.V. Mattingley whose special interest was the dental condition of the Aborigine people. Fish's thinking about the causes of periodontal disease was significantly influenced by this work. Mattingley's son, K.V. Mattingley, wrote about his father in an interesting book, 'Dentist on a Camel', in which his father's contact with Fish is described.

The years 1924-34 were possibly the most crowded in Fish's life. In notes written about thirty years later he lists some thirty projects in which he was engaged in that decade. In April 1932 Fish was involved in two very important matters that came before the Medical Committee at the RDH.

The first related to the presence of female students. Applications for entry to RDH had dropped. This may have been due to the economic depression, but the demonstrators felt that " the presence of female students is probably a definite deterrent to the entry of male students." No explanation of how the young ladies caused this negative effect is given. Did they distract the young gentlemen from their studies, or was it that the presence of women tended to lower the tone of a severely masculine and chauvinist profession? The matter was taken so seriously that it was referred, not to a sub-committee but to the Board of Management. In June the Dean stated that "in the best interests of the school women should be excluded", and at the meeting of July 7th. Dr. Fish moved "that women students be no longer admitted to the school, provided that nothing in this resolution should prejudice the position of women already admitted." The resolution was passed unanimously. Was Fish simply complying with the Board's wishes, or did the resolution truly reflect his view of women at that time?

This antipathy to the presence of women had manifested itself in earlier years, when there was considerable resistance to the introduction of dental nurses and dental assistants. This resistance was also displayed in the columns of the British Dental Journal, and it was not until 1929 that nurses were employed at the RDH.

Also in April of 1932 Fish proposed that a department be set up for the "the treatment of periodontal diseases", and Professor Stobie agreed. Fish suggested that such a department should be in charge of an Honorary Assistant Dental Surgeon for one session a week, together with a half time demonstrator to attend each afternoon at a salary of £250 per year. This suggestion met with no objection and a sub-committee was appointed to work out the details and to be presented to the Board of Management. Thus, in that year Fish established the first periodontal department in Britain. As part of its activity four student dressers each month carried out scalings, and senior students were made responsible for "more complicated treatment." Gingivectomy was on the agenda.

In 1932 two important figures appeared on the part-time staff of the RDH. B.F. Fickling became a house surgeon in the prosthetics department, and Robert Bradlaw who was to play, in the opinion of many, as important a role in dentistry as Fish himself, was appointed as a demonstrator and joined Fish in the research laboratory. Ben Fickling, who was to become an influential Chairman of the Medical Committee, took charge of the periodontal department when Fish left the R.D.H, and obtaining his FRCS on the way, supervised the growth of the department until it became a university department under his successor, A.B.Wade.

The Hale laboratory with its animal house on the roof of the hospital was a hive of activity, its work well respected abroad. The eminent teacher at Columbia University School of Dentistry, C.F. Bodecker, wrote to Fish in January 1931, "I was very pleased to hear from you and to note the atmosphere of intense energy and active work." Some feeling of the atmosphere in the laboratory is painted in a letter from Singapore from Aubrey Stonyer, a former research assistant. In March 1933 he wrote, "The reading of your book brought back many pleasant memories of happy days in the Dental Hospital, again I can see the dogs, monkeys, India ink, methylated blue and piles of photographs, busy, happy days, full of interest, with work made a pleasure by a kind and considerate chief...."

Lilian Lindsey, then Honorary Librarian to the BDA wrote, "your work is quoted in every country where the subject of metabolism and the histology of enamel and dentine is treated."

In 1933 Fish was awarded his Doctorate of Science by University College London where the work was completed. Congratulations poured in from all over the world when his book, " An experimental investigation of enamel, dentine and the dental pulp", was published.

Even before the publication of his research, Fish had been made an Honorary member of the Dental association of Vienna in 1931, and of the Spanish Dental Association in 1932. His reputation was further enhanced when the first edition of his book, " Principles of Denture Prosthesis" appeared and was an immediate sell-out.

Some years later his portrait was painted in doctoral robes by Francis Hodge. It is a traditional, formal but sympathetic rendering of the man, in his forties but still looking young, a considerable success, high forehead, serious, but betraying some humour, perhaps at finding himself in this happy situation. As an elderly lady, when talking about her second husband, Hazel frequently describes his bright blue eyes, his impish sense of humour and liking for practical jokes.

Hodge also painted Hilda's portrait, and a sitting at his studio provided the only occasion when Hilda and Hazel met each other. Some years after their marriage Hazel painted a much more informal portrait of Fish seated at his desk with papers scattered about. This portrait now hangs on the first landing of the British Dental Association headquarters at Wimpole Street.

Despite the productivity of the research department and Fish's success, the department hobbled from one difficulty to another, even though it received a donation of £250 from an old student, F.R.Moser. Fish became increasingly impatient with the situation, and in 1935 the Board of Management noted that Dr. Fish appeared to be responsible for incurring expenditure without the sanction of the Board.

In June 1936 an anonymous letter to the Board of Management reported that the research department had been enlarged without any proper costing and now had an overdraft of £880. "Research", this letter continued, "although desirable and advantageous, was not a direction in which funds for charitable purposes can be utilised." Further, it said that public knowledge that operations were carried out on live animals would be prejudicial to the Hospital, and the Hospital should divorce itself from any liability or connection with the Research Department.

Earlier that year the sub-committee on research had reported that, "further difficulties had arisen in the Research Department and that no more dogs be kept there." It resolved, "that research be confined to such research as is possible without animals."

In July the Board of Management unanimously decided that, "after December 1936 no research should be carried out which involved experiments on animals other than rats, mice and guinea pigs."

The facts behind this decision are something of a tragi-comedy. A dog, while being exercised on the roof of the RDH had fallen to its death in Leicester Square. The dog was part of Fish's enquiry into changes in bone metabolism related to nutritional deficiencies. Animals in captivity are more prone to rickets than animals in the wild, and dogs' bones are especially prone to rickets from disuse. Daily exercise is essential, especially when they are kept in cages for most of the time. The presence of rickets in dogs on an apparently adequate diet, including a good supply of Vitamin D, would certainly confuse any observations of other metabolic changes.

Fish's late awareness of this complication is noted in his hand on an envelope containing photographs and a report of the dogs' dietary regime. Fish wrote, "A bit of the Vitamin D story - that cost me dear!." and "It showed you get rickets in large young dogs on full doses of Vitamin D if you do not exercise them .... and cure it by exercise without Vitamin D - very naughty."

One can imagine his immediate reaction to this omission. A porter must have been ordered to attend to the matter of daily exercise, and perhaps a moment of inattention, pause to light a cigarette up on a windy roof, allowed a dog to wander over the edge.

The photographs themselves are intriguing. In the report Fish details the diet of the puppies from birth. He writes that they were born at a veterinary surgeon's practice and exercised in a concrete yard, but the photographs of the poor, bowlegged and rachitic puppies were taken in a garden with crazy paving. In one photograph the dogs are in the charge of woman in a raincoat (only the lower part of the figure shows), possibly Hilda, and in the others being looked after by an adolescent boy in a suit with long trousers, more than likely Fish's son James. This possibility fits in with the fact of Fish's inclination to work at home. Maybe he conscripted the family to his research activity; it would not be surprising in someone so driven by his work. By this time Fish and his family had moved away from Sevenoaks to nearby Hildenborough where they had a large house with a 5-acre garden. Fish had bought for his son James, then in his early 'teens, an old Morris car, only chassis and engine, which James raced around the garden.

The publicity surrounding the bizarre death of the dog must have appalled everyone, especially the laymen on the Board of Management. Fish must have been severely embarrassed, and he probably suffered enough envy and hostility from the Medical Committee to evoke a strong response. It was the beginning of the end of his connection with the RDH .

Further problems for Fish stemmed from a debate about his grant from the MRC, which, because of his conflict with Mrs. May Mellanby, looked with disfavour on both himself and his research. Unfortunately Edward Mellanby, May's husband, was now secretary to the MRC. On the other hand, the Dental Board respected Fish and his work, which they were very much in favour of supporting. A letter dated 19 October 1936, from M. Murray, a colleague of Mrs. Mellanby's at Bedford College, to the MRC explains that, "there is general agreement of The Dental Caries Committee that the grant to Dr.E.W. Fish and Mr. Ross should be reduced" but such a procedure would be politically unwise....probably against the wishes of the Dental Board. "The MRC agreed with this resolution, but as no representative of the Dental Board happened to be present at that particular meeting of the Dental Caries Committee, no decision was taken. Several letters were exchanged between members of the committee, and finally a compromise was reached on the basis of the fact that the grant of £100 to the biochemist, Dr. Paul Pincus, who was resigning his post at the Hale laboratory, could be transferred to Fish. This allowed Fish's grant from the MRC to be reduced by that amount. It was decided that this would be so until Fish started his research work at St. Mary's Hospital and applied for a new grant, when " the Council (MRC) might not be able to continue its support at the same rate."

Both the form and the cost of Fish's work were the source of difficulty for the Board of Management, especially as the disagreement with the Mellanbys had soured the relationship between the RDH and the MRC. On the 22nd. October 1936 a special sub-committee met to report back to the Board of Management on the future of the research department. Professor Stobie was in the chair, attended only by Mr. Turner and Dr. Fish.

The minutes report that; "The Sub-Committee first considered the scheme of maintaining a small Research Department upon the lines suggested by Mr. Turner, carrying out the following research work:- human and lower animal histology, the results of malnutrition in such animals as rats, mice and guinea pigs and on the pathogenicity of bacteria. However, such a department would prove to be impractical purely on financial grounds."

Next Fish put forward his scheme, whereby he and his co-workers would continue to work in the Department, but within the limits laid down by the Board of Management. He further produced figures in support of his claim that such a department would be financially practicable for a period of one year.

The following is Dr. Fish's conception of the financial out-look for the year in question:-

Assets			Liabilities	
A. Paid by the Hospital for pathology	150		*A.* Overhead expenses	260
B. Gift from Messrs. Reckitt	25			
C. Gift from Mr.E.W. Meyerstein	300			
	475			**260**
D. Grants from the M.R.C. to Dr. Fish and his Colleagues.	722		*B.* Wages	500
			C. Materials	X
	£1,197			**£760 + X**

This leaves £437 to cover the item X and any contingencies that might arise.

"The existing Research department enjoys an income from investments of £50 drawn from the Hale Investment of £1,000 and the Moser Endowment of £250. At the present time it is probable that the Hale Investment will be realised to liquidate the existing overdraft. Dr. Fish proposes that the school should take over the existing Hale investment, if such a transfer is possible, on the termination of the present Research Department in December 1936 and liquidate the overdraft of funds which it may have available for investment."

"The Sub-Committee therefore conclude that Dr. Fish's scheme would be financially practicable for one year, assuming that the Medical Research Council continue their grants and that Mr. Meyerstein includes his gift of £300."

It was proposed, seconded and resolved to recommend to the Board of Management :-

" That the School takes over the Research Department for one year from 1st. January, 1937, that Dr. Fish's offer to guarantee the department against any financial loss on the running of the department be accepted in writing , and that in the event of any part of the income of the department ceasing, the whole question of the existence of the department be reconsidered immediately."

It was also agreed that the accounts of the department be kept strictly in accordance with the system approved by the School Auditors and be submitted each month to the Finance Committee for payment.

Fish's days of independence in running the Research Department were over. Not only that, his guarantee of financial support could mean a substantial commitment to support research of little personal interest to him. Furthermore he had already established a worthwhile connection with St. Mary's Hospital, and could be more of his own master there in both clinical and research work.

On 17th. June of the following year the Board of Management received Fish's letter of resignation from his post as Honorary Dental Surgeon. He stated that he proposed to move his research work to St. Mary's Hospital. The Board decided to accept his resignation with sincere regret and thanked him for his many valuable services to the hospital and school. On the 1st. July 1937 the Medical Committee unanimously resolved "that this committee thanks E. W. Fish very much for his many services, and regrets his resignation."

When Fish departed the atmosphere at the Hale laboratory became less than happy. The directorship was taken on again by the now elderly J.G. Turner, but with not too much success. The biochemist, Paul Pincus, who had worked with Fish, regularly complained to Dean Stobie, that he could not work with people, "who have had no experience in research or laboratory work of any kind beyond that met in the usual dental training." Pincus also complained of his working conditions. It seems that when he arrived in the morning the concrete floor of his room was still wet from the cleaners. Dr. Pincus soon left for the Department of Biochemistry at the University of Melbourne.

Despite the problems that he had encountered, Fish could only look back on his twelve years at the RDH with satisfaction. In looking back over the years of intense activity from 1924-34, Fish listed some thirty enterprises in which he had been engaged. These included his research on the cardiovascular effects of local anaesthetic solutions, the circulation of lymph in dentine, the loss of calcium salts from dentine, the reaction of the pulp to injury of dentine, infection in bone, stabilising factors in full denture construction, and many other topics. He had translated himself from the relative obscurity of Sevenoaks into a figure of international standing within his profession.

Despite the fact that the RDH had been admitted as a School of London University since 1911, at the time of the 1956 UGC visitation, after Stobie had retired, the Honorary Dental Surgeons and Assistant Dental Surgeons, all part-time, of whom the Dean was one, ran the school more or less as had been the case since its foundation. The advent of the National Health Service in 1948 boosted the clinical activity of the Hospital side, but change in the undergraduate curriculum was slow, research activity was limited, and there were few senior full-time academic appointments. Following the Quinquennial Visit of the University Grants Committee to the Royal Dental Hospital (RDH) in 1956, Sir Keith Murray, Chairman of the UGC, declared, "Of all the schools visited, and indeed, one might say of all the University institutions so far visited throughout the country, the Royal Dental Hospital School of Dental Surgery was the least satisfactory." This was regarded by many as scarcely a fair judgement, for as Smith and Cottell point out, in 1955 the Dean had asked H.M. Pickard, Reader in Conservative Dentistry, former student and a good friend of Fish, plus Alan Mack, Assistant Director of the Prosthetic Department, Bryan Wade, Assistant Director of the Department of Periodontology, and D.P. Walther, Reader in Orthodontics, to reform the teaching programme. This they did with considerable success, but without Fish who was in any case over sixty. The following years were to demonstrate their considerable success in bringing teaching and research activity at the RDH, largely under the full-time Dean, the pathologist Professor R.B.Lucas, to a level which even the workers at Guy's Hospital and the London came to envy.

Alas, thirty years later, following a "rationalisation" of London hospitals and their schools, the RDH was absorbed into Guy's Hospital, finally to disappear altogether except as a piece of history.

Fish did return to the RDH, and to the Hampton Hale Laboratory on many occasions, and in the preface to his last book, 'Surgical Pathology of the Mouth', published in 1948, and essentially a compilation of his research and thinking, he writes, "It is not possible to say how much the author owes to his old colleagues at the John Hampton Hale Research Laboratory ... they are all gratefully remembered." One wonders how his continuing presence on the staff might have influenced the future of the institution, but once he was elected in 1939 to the Dental Board of the United Kingdom, his efforts were bent on improving the reputation of his profession as a worthy speciality of medicine.

Chapter 8

THE MELLANBY STORY

In 1930, on the occasion of the British Dental Association's Jubilee celebrations, Mrs. (later Lady) May Mellanby Sc.D., MA (Cantab),was made an honorary member of the association in recognition of " her contribution to dental science."

Mrs. Mellanby was a physiologist who worked tirelessly throughout her life, mainly in the field of nutrition, and for many years concentrated on the role of nutrition in relation to the development of the dentition and the causation of dental caries. Her research work was regarded as so important that in the 1935 special issue of the Dental Magazine and Oral Topics, which included a 'Dental Panorama' celebrating 25 years of the reign of King George V, the first item for the year 1930 was the Medical Research Council's publication of the "First part of Mrs. May Mellanby's report on 'Diet and the Teeth'". The second part of that report was duly noted as an important event of 1931.

Born May Tweedy in 1883, eleven years before Wilfred Fish, and from a well-to-do family, she was educated at Hampstead and Bromley High Schools before going to Girton College, Cambridge, where she took the Natural Science Tripos. She went on to teach and carry out research at Bedford College for Women at a time of struggle for women's emancipation. The suffragettes, Emmeline Pankhurst, and her daughters, Sylvia, Christabel (later Dame) and Adela, had initiated direct-action and hunger strikes. Many wealthy women supported the movement, borrowing their maid's clothes to go unrecognised to meetings at Caxton Hall. Girton and Somerville College, Oxford, provided a fertile soil for the movement, which May Mellanby could not ignore, even if she disagreed with the radical nature of the movement. The biological sciences offered advancement for women long before physics offered the same opportunities. Despite the early example of Marie Curie, double Nobel laureate, universities were resistant to the appointment of women teachers of physics.

Cambridge did not award a Ph.D. in physics to a woman until 1926, but women working in biology fared better. It was a time for opportunity for someone as energetic and ambitious as May Mellanby.

In 1914 at the age of thirty-two, and holding the post of Research Scholar at Bedford College, she married the distinguished physiologist Edward Mellanby, two years her junior, and childless, they collaborated in research throughout the rest of their lives together.

Mellanby (later Sir Edward) is noted for his research on nutrition, the role of vitamins and the deficiency diseases, in particular rickets. He established that the main cause of the disease was deficiency of a fat-soluble vitamin, which came to be known as Vitamin D. He also demonstrated in his animal experiments that light enhanced the effectiveness of Vitamin D in the diet. It was a common observation that where the heavily polluted air of the great cities, centres of the manufacturing industries, blocked out sunlight, and where infants were kept indoors, the incidence of rickets was higher than in the countryside. We now know that Vitamin D is obtained primarily from the action of ultra-violet light on the skin, but then nutrition was the focus of attention.

In 1920 Mellanby was appointed to the Chair in Pharmacology at the University of Sheffield, and was elected FRS in 1925. He became Chairman of the League of Nations Nutrition and Vitamin Standardisation Commission, and in 1937 was knighted. Subsequently he received a coveted medical accolade when he became an Honorary Physician to King George VI. This honour was conferred on distinguished doctors after they had retired.

One of his major roles was as Secretary to the Medical Research Council to which he was appointed in 1933. This was an extremely powerful position from which to influence decisions as to which research the MRC should support. He was a man with a strong personality, and it is reported that he could be very brusque; and " he said what he thought, apparently without consideration for the feelings of the person to whom he was speaking". One can imagine that he did not suffer gladly those he thought fools, and it seems possible that he would reject applications for work that did not fit in with his own scientific views. However he gave his wife all necessary backing in her research, which might be regarded as a corollary of his own.

The Mellanbys were highly respected members of the scientific community, and May Mellanby was a friend of the Fabian Socialists, Beatrice and Sidney Webb, who in 1913 launched the left-wing magazine, The New Statesman. Despite her strong socialist convictions Beatrice Webb did not approve of the militant feminist movement, and perhaps in that she and May Mellanby were of like mind. May Mellanby was also a friend of Margaret and Ramsay MacDonald, who became the first Labour Prime Minister of Britain in 1924, to be re-elected in 1929, and again in 1931 as leader of the National Government. The Mellanbys had easy access to the levers of power and influence.

When Mrs. Mellanby started her research work on nutrition, three vitamins were known. These were an 'Antiscorbutic', 'Water-soluble B or antineuritic', and 'Fat-soluble A' (this turned out to be a complex of Vitamins A, D and E), on which her work, like her husband's, was focussed. Her dedication was total, and the volume of her work on the influence of nutrition on the development and disease of the dentition, starting around 1917, is enormous.

Although various investigations were carried out concurrently, her work falls into three groups: the incidence of defectively formed and decayed teeth in children; the influence of nutrition on the development of animal teeth; the influence of nutrition on children's teeth. In this work, her dental model was J.Howard Mummery CBE, FRCS, who held a "unique position as the final court of appeal on matters of dental histology and pathology". His pioneer work on the nerve supply of dentine required immensely careful sectioning of both hard and soft tissues to avoid distortion, something previous workers had been unable to achieve. This achievement is all the more impressive when one realises that most of this work was carried out in a laboratory at his home. He would attend meetings with his slides in his pocket hoping that an opportunity would arise when he could show them. It is said that after repeated manifestations of his colleagues' disinterest in his slides, he stopped going to scientific meetings altogether. His prestige was enhanced by the fact that he had seven papers published in the Philosophical Transactions of the Royal Society. However he, like Fish, was not to be elected to a Fellowship.

In all her work Mrs. Mellanby's thinking followed a distinct line; nutrition affects the structure of teeth, structure influences the vulnerability of teeth to decay, and nutrition can thus affect the progress of dental decay. In this her thinking parallels Edward Mellanby's work on rickets, in which both teeth and bone are formed defectively because of failure in calcification. In describing one of his studies on the role of fat-soluble A in meat in puppies' diet, Mellanby states, "The action of meat is undoubtedly inhibitory in nature (to rickets), and when fifty grams of meat are given will almost prevent rickets in a growing puppy. Meat has a stimulating action on the growth of puppies far beyond its fat-soluble A content, so also it appears now that the anti-rachitic action of meat is in a greater measure than any fat-soluble A it is reputed to contain."

The idea that structure influences the prevalence of decay was the source of most controversy. Mrs. Mellanby defined normal dentine as being free of interglobular spaces, and their presence a sign of defective formation. Also, she claimed that where calcospherites had not completely coalesced this represented slight hypoplasia. She studied hypoplasia in the puppies used by Edward Mellanby, as well as in other animals, before extending her observations to children. She examined 1,036 deciduous teeth in 6-9 year-olds in care homes, and found that 85.6% were defective and carious. She concluded that "there is a direct relationship between structure and caries, those badly formed most carious; those well formed less carious ... Structure is probably controlled by dietetic factors." She examined these teeth both clinically, and by microscopic examination of ground sections, and came to the conclusion that the data obtained macroscopically, as in the clinical situation, was fallacious. The dentist was therefore an imperfect witness. Only microscopic examination revealed those otherwise undetected defects in calcification, and some dietary problem, most specifically lack of Vitamin D, but also an excess of cereals (an idea of her husband's in relation to rickets), produced the defects. When Professor W. H. Gilmour at Liverpool, the holder of the first Chair of Dental Surgery in the country, stated that, "He could substantiate the view that in gross hypoplasia caries does not occur more frequently," Mrs. Mellanby asserted that she was not referring to the kind of hypoplasia seen by dentists, but to " a second type of hypoplasia less evident to the naked eye." Perhaps she was then informed that Sir Frank Colyer, the doyen of dental teachers at that time, had reported that in many great apes in the wild considerable hypoplasia occurred in the complete absence of caries, because later, she appeared to be less dogmatic when she asked the rhetorical question, " Why is the relationship between the structure of the teeth and the incidence of caries not absolute? Is it partly because fully erupted teeth, whatever their structure, have some power of altering their resistance to caries, and if so what is the mechanism which controls this resistance?" This notion of the tooth's capacity to alter its resistance to caries produced even more controversy.

Colyer was a great traveller. It was a time when the affluent with an army of porters, could explore exotic areas of the world, and bag their portion of animals in the wild. He travelled extensively in S.America, the Amazon, the East Indies and Africa, and so huge was his spoil that he could present the museum of the BDA with 4,000 specimens. From sixty species of animal he made 280 ground sections of tooth tissue, and found poorly mineralised enamel in almost all animals other than the macaques. Today we realise that the quality of mineralisation cannot be assessed by the optical microscope, and that more sophisticated techniques, such as micro-radiography, need to be used. However, Mrs. Mellanby was dogmatic that her assessment of the quality of tooth structure was correct, and could not be diverted from her theory of the important connection between structure and caries prevalence.

In the Lancet, December 1918, and in her contribution to a publication, 'The Gateway to Health', she writes, " few will deny that much dental trouble is caused by the changed diet of man, as the result of civilization, but the question that still remains to a great extent unanswered is: what are the dietetic factors, the presence or absence of which are responsible for the poor structure and liability to decay of the teeth of civilized man and of many animals in captivity?"

"Diet in respect of the teeth must be considered from two points of view:-

1. The part played by the foodstuffs while still in the mouth
2. The part played by these substances after absorption from the alimentary canal into the blood."

She continued, "The first of these problems is no doubt important, but I question whether it is of such consequence as some authorities think; the second on the other hand seems to me fundamental...". (It is interesting to note that in his theory of periodontal disease, Fish also compared 'primitive' and 'civilized' man, but took the view that the state of the oral tissues was critical to an understanding of periodontal disease. The end of the nineteenth century saw the start of considerable interest in anthropology, and in so-called 'primitive' people.)

In a paper given in November 1919 to the British Society for the Study of Orthodontics, Mrs. Mellanby presented her experimental evidence demonstrating the influence of a special dietetic factor on the development of the teeth and jaws.

In her paper, she stated that Calcium cannot be used by the tissues "for the proper construction of normal teeth and bone unless fat-soluble A, or something with a similar distribution is also present." She decried the fact that there was so much cereal in the diet instead of meat, and pointed out that in Poland and Austria teeth were very defective because during the war the diet was deficient in milk, eggs, animal fats, and other foods containing fat-soluble A.

In her lecture she went on to quote a writer in the Lancet (not named) who stated, "Experience has taught me that there is no royal road to the prevention of dental caries. To believe that our nation will alter its diet to save its teeth is chimerical. The chief safeguards are cleanliness, inspection and early treatment." To which she responds, "The origin of many of our dental defects is, possibly largely dietetic and that the factor at fault is very definite in its action.........If my work and its application to human beings is correct one important cause of unsound teeth and poor growth of the jaws is very well defined and does not involve the use of that hopeless expression, 'defective hygiene'."

This pejorative reference to defective hygiene is almost certainly aimed at the distinguished Scottish dental scientist, James Sim Wallace. Wallace obtained his MB in Glasgow in 1890 before he was twenty-one, and after being a ship's doctor took an LDS at the Royal Dental Hospital. He wrote an MD thesis on Nitrous Oxide anaesthesia, and then in 1900 obtained the first D.Sc. in the country for a thesis confined to a dental subject, " The Cause and Prevention of Decay in Teeth."

He was a man before his time, and became lecturer in preventive dentistry at King's College. It is said that his premises for his doctrine of prevention were, "first find the cause of the trouble, next remove it," and "thou shalt finish a meal with some fibrous and detergent food." Then in an article in the journal, The Child, April 1911, in which he details a day's menu for children, he wrote, "decay in teeth, or dental caries as it is called, and those diseases resulting from the unhygienic state of the mouth....when the above rules ...cannot be observed, some attempt should be made to clean the crevices between the teeth with a small toothbrush, but if it is advisable to have children taken regularly to the dentist from the age of three onwards every six months."

If Sim Wallace was the unnamed writer in the Lancet, Mrs. Mellanby would have dismissed his clinical observations as empirical and uncontrolled, and therefore not scientific. It was a very good example of the frequent antagonism between clinicians and research workers, which Fish was to decry; indeed one of the last letters he wrote before he died, was on this very topic. Mrs. Mellanby's criticisms of dental research was also representative of the medical establishment's attitude to dentists and their research.

Mrs. Mellanby went on to compare the dentition of puppies on a variety of diets, with or without cod-liver oil, Vitamin D, egg yolk, a little or a lot of cereal, etc. and concluded that, "even with Calcium and Phosphorus sound teeth and jaws do not develop without some other nutritional factors being present which allow those elements (Ca and P) to be retained in the body, and which promote their disposition in the growing body as Calcium phosphate."

In commenting on other opinions, she stated that, "recent research confirms Miller's chemo-parasitic theory of the origin of dental caries, but my experimental work on puppies and the statistical investigations recorded here seem to indicate that this side of the problem is comparatively unimportant.... When however the teeth are badly formed .... Then the presence of bacteria and food debris in the crevices of the teeth, the hydrogen and calcium ion concentrations of the fluid bathing the teeth, and other conditions in the mouth, are undoubtedly of great significance in dental disease."

Mrs. Mellanby was so certain of her case that she extended her studies to controlled experiments on the diet of children in institutions.

As stated some of Edward Mellanby's research appeared to indicate that cereals contained a factor antagonistic to Vitamin D, and therefore interfering with calcification, to produced defectively formed teeth. So Mrs. Mellanby divided 32 children, average age 7.5 years, into three dietary groups. Group A received a diet rich in vitamins and without cereals; group B had oatmeal, very little egg, no cod-liver oil, and less milk than group A. Group C was placed in an intermediary position, and on 'an ordinary hospital diet.'

The children were watched over for seven months, new carious cavities were counted and teeth assessed for changes in hardening or softening by simple probing.

New teeth becoming carious were 0.65 per child in group A; 2.8 in group B, and 1.45 in group C. Hardening and softening followed the expected and similar pattern.

In summary the results confirmed her belief was that there

was a definite association between tooth structure and the susceptibility to dental caries. Lack of calcium and phosphorus was the cause, and a diet rich in these substances even after the formation and eruption of the teeth, would affect their resistance to caries.

The Mellanbys references to the idea that there was something in cereals which interferes with calcification, seems to hark back to the "lactic acid theory" of the cause of rickets. This theory maintained that lactic acid was generated in excess by the fermentation of starchy food imperfectly digested. By its absorption into the circulation the acid united with the lime of the bone forming a soluble salt which was removed from the system. Alas, the theory did not explain the defects in all the other tissues.

Mrs. Mellanby may also have been influenced by the apparent correlation between the prevalence of rickets, hypoplastic teeth and caries, and the difference in diet of the poor and the more affluent. The poor ate little meat and a great deal of carbohydrate in bread and potatoes, while the better-off ate less carbohydrate and more meat. What was certainly not taken into account was the difference in environment of the poor and better-off. The urban poor lived in small, dark and crowded dwellings, and the sun was filtered through the heavily polluted atmosphere of industrial cities. Today we know that sunshine is an essential ingredient of the synthesis of Vitamin D, but that was not yet known.

A report of the Mellanby research appeared in the British Medical Journal of August 1924, as well as in the British Dental Journal. The latter report was followed by a critical comment which began, "We make these comments in no carping spirit, but with the desire of elucidating the full significance of this interesting and important paper."

The anonymous writer goes on to question whether observations on puppies can be applied to man. But the main criticism rested on Mrs. Mellanby's assumption that calcified tissues are subject to metabolic changes after their formation, that enamel can be affected by diet after it is formed, and that the quality of secondary dentine produced as a response to caries depended on diet, and might therefore by good diet correct caries. The writer commented, "in the children examined the teeth present or which erupted during the investigation, must have been fully calcified long before ..so far as the primary calcification of the teeth is concerned the research does not prove that it is dependent on the vitamin content of the diet.. . a good diet might result in well formed secondary dentine in poorly calcified teeth and act as a barrier to the spread of caries." Further, " the power of the dentine to react to a stimulus through the pulp has long been a commonplace, but it had been assumed that this reaction can only occur after there is a breach of the enamel."

Was Wallace the writer of this comment? There is no record, but there were many other dissenting voices.

The Profession's Response

Most dentists who wished to carry out research had no resources and depended upon observations that they made in their patients' mouths. A few were able to make ground sections, but without financial support such activity was very limited. Unfortunately, because of Edward Mellanby's influence at the MRC any work that did not appear to support his wife's point of view would not be funded.

However Evelyn Sprawson, who was to become Sub-Dean and Director of Dental Studies at the London Hospital Dental School, and held Sim Wallace in high regard, was dentist to the Dr. Barnardo's Homes, and therefore had ready access to a community of children. This allowed him to carry out studies of caries prevalence in children, albeit in a smaller scale investigation than Mrs. Mellanby's. Also he recruited a teacher of chemistry to carry out a study of the chemical composition of enamel. His conclusions seemed to be confused. Like Wallace he held that "freedom from caries depends largely on the physical character of their foods", but he also stated, "it has been shown that deficiency of either Vitamin A or B, or C or D separately, causes errors in calcification... which apparently predisposed them to caries ." On the other hand, " Vitamin D has been shown conclusively to be no preventive of caries"; also "my own investigations showed that immunity to caries was produced even when cereals...were frequently taken."

His explanation of that immunity lay in his conviction that it could be provided by drinking raw rather than pasteurised milk, and his research concentrated on its proof.

The doyen dental teacher, Sir Frank Colyer, regarded Mrs. Mellanby as a "harmful intruder in her thinking about caries."

The response to Mrs. Mellanby's assertion that not only the state of calcification of teeth after their formation, but also that the course of the carious process could be altered by diet, met with a two-pronged attack from the dental profession. Both clinicians and dental researchers reacted with some vigour.

The most forceful rebuttal from a clinician came from Robert Weaver, a former student of Gilmour in Liverpool. Weaver was the first person with a dental qualification (he had an MD as well) to be appointed to the medical staff of the Board of Education. In a long and distinguished career in public health work, for which as the Senior Medical Officer to the Ministry of Education, he was awarded CBE, he had a considerable influence on promoting the dental health of schoolchildren.

It was said of him that "he loved a good argument and was certainly no fence-sitter over important issues." This opinion of Weaver was confirmed by his article in the BDJ, "Diet and the Teeth", written as a response to the publication of the third part of Mrs. Mellanby's 1934 MRC report on that subject, and the adoption of the report by the National Dental Services Committee and Representative Board of the BDA.

Their approval of the Mellanby work was expressed in the following words. "The Association is impressed by the results of the investigations into the causation of dental caries and it recommends that over and above routine curative treatment, instruction to correct errors in diet and, when indicated, the prescribing of therapeutic remedies to promote a higher resistance to dental caries.... Should be included in the scope of the Dental Health Service."

Weaver's general comment was that, "Although this

recommendation does not indicate specifically the remedies...
it will be generally interpreted as an endorsement of Mrs.
Mellanby's recommendations." His detailed attack on her
theories was much more to the point. He pointed out that her
findings were not in harmony with many facts:-

1. Although Mrs. Mellanby could produce structural defects in
   the developing teeth of puppies, she could not produce dental
   caries , therefore some other influence must be at work.
2. Her methods of assessing structure were unsound, and in
   assessing caries she had aggregated cases of slight caries
   with those with no caries.
3. While one would expect dental defects in developing teeth
   caused by defects in diet to be symmetrical, caries was often
   asymmetrical on opposite sides of the mouth.
4. There was a greater liability to caries in pulpless than in
   vital teeth.
5. There was no evidence that children with severe rickets had
   more severe caries.
6. It had not been established that the resistance of a tooth to
   caries can be raised or lowered by diet
7. There is a different liability of different surfaces of teeth to
   caries.
8. In sunlit South Africa, New Zealand and Australia, rickets is
   practically unknown, but teeth still suffer caries.

Weaver concluded, "There is a very good reason why a
nutritional theory should not be adopted in place of an
environmental theory before the latter has been conclusively
proved to be wrong... an environmental theory says that if the
teeth are not subject to the action of acid they will not become
carious - an argument which is easily understood. How can a
tooth, however well formed, resist an attack which is primarily
chemical, what is there in the teeth which can prevent acid from
dissolving the enamel of those teeth with which it remains in
contact? Is it conceivable that, as fast as the enamel is
decalcified, the vitality or "resistance" of the tooth effects a
recalcification?"

Following his publications in the BDJ, Weaver presented a paper, "The relative importance of various factors in the aetiology of caries" at the 9th. International Dental Congress of the F.D.I. in Vienna in August 1936. His criticisms of the Mellanby theory to an international audience met with an immediate and powerful response from both Mellanbys. Mrs. Mellanby wrote to Weaver that people in Vienna thought he spoke in an official capacity and that "you appear to have misread or misinterpreted many statements made in the reports of my investigation." Edward Mellanby's intervention was more lethal. He complained to Sir Arthur MacNulty, head of the Board of Education, for which government department Weaver worked, and asked, was Weaver expressing his own personal views or did they represent the views of the department? Many people assumed the latter, and Mellanby hoped that this was not the case.

MacNulty was quick to assure Mellanby that Weaver's paper expressed his personal opinion, and wrote to Weaver for his assurance on this account. Weaver replied immediately that the paper expressed his own views, not those of the department. He also wrote to Mrs. Mellanby , expressing his sincere regret that anyone should think he was expressing himself in his official capacity, "as Sir Arthur has told me that, whilst I hold my official position, it is undesirable for me to engage in scientific controversy." Weaver saw the red light and resigned from his secretary position of the International Oral Hygiene Commission of the Federation Dentaire Internationale. This move must have given Mrs. Mellanby a twinge of conscience, because in January 1937 (the year her husband was knighted) she wrote to Spencer L. Rowles, then treasurer of the FDI, denying that Weaver's "withdrawal from 'scientific controversy' is in some way instigated by myself."

It is illuminating of the Mellanby's personal relationship that she felt the need to write to a friend that "I have often had to suffer Sir Walter Fletcher's and my husband's indiscretions", and "I have all along tried to curtail Sir Walter Fletcher and my husband's ardour over my work." The episode demonstrates Edward Mellanby's power and influence, as well as his attitude to his wife and her work. They were, after all, a married couple of their time.

The medical establishment and initially even some dentists, accepted the Mellanby theories. Mrs. Mellanby's research had the support of the Medical Research Council. Both Mellanbys were held in great esteem by the medical and dental establishment, and the widest possible publicity was given to their views. The Mellanby theory about the origin of caries was treated with unquestioning respect. In fact the Mellanby influence crossed the Atlantic. A study carried out by the Murray and Leonie Guggenheim Dental Clinic compared caries prevalence in children in their own homes with those in foster homes on a controlled diet, and concluded that caries was the result not only of local causes, but also of defective nutrition. This was as late as 1941.

Inevitably the pharmaceutical business recognised an opportunity for profit in Mrs. Mellanby's ideas. A product called 'Calfos', a "preparation of the unaltered basic constituent of bone from which fat, sinew and water-soluble protein have been removed" was put on the market in tablet form. It was recommended to be taken during pregnancy, lactation, in any cases of malnutrition where Calcium and Phosphorus need to be supplemented, including rickets, chilblains and dental caries. A supporting booklet explained the aetiology of dental caries, citing the work of Mellanby, Dr. J.D. King, a dental researcher with an MRC grant, and others. By the use of "generous therapeutic doses... the number and size of fillings.. will be reduced or the need for conservation even abolished."

So well promoted was this product that the London County Council, an organisation that often referred to Mrs. Mellanby about dental matters, organised a survey which seems to have been so badly organised that the statistician, a Dr. Sinclair, found difficulty in coming to a firm conclusion, but did indicate that the claims made for Calfos could not be substantiated.

These arguments, which had started around 1924 at the beginning of Fish's research on tooth tissue, rumbled on for years. In October 1936, Fish wrote to Sir David Munro, Director of the MRC, "there is very little possibility of obtaining a carious second premolar with immune neighbours ... this suggests that structure is never a sufficiently potent factor to save a tooth from destruction if its environment is wrong."

The Mellanby theories were widely known, the BDJ and BMJ were read in the USA, and Rudolf Kronfeld, a student of Gottlieb's, a distinguished research worker, and author of "Histopathology of the Teeth and their Surrounding Structures," and one of the many who found refuge from Hitler in the USA, wrote, "It has been said that the quality of prenatal calcification may influence the caries incidence in deciduous teeth. This claim is based upon a disregard of the anatomic facts. Caries always begins at the surface of the enamel, which with the exception of the incisal portion of the incisors consists of postnatally formed enamel. The highest incidence of caries in deciduous teeth lies in the proximo-gingival level of all teeth, and in the occlusal fissures of the deciduous molars. Thus, it can be seen, by simple observation, that caries in deciduous teeth always begins in postnatal enamel, and its incidence cannot be affected by any prenatal quality or modification of calcification."

Mrs. Mellanby's answer to the many criticisms of her caries research was an elegant piece of obfuscation. "It is obvious that both the exciting and predisposing causes of caries are complex, and that there may be many subsidiary factors, including some unknown nutritional factors, the physical and chemical nature of the food, the variety of micro-organisms , and heredity, all of which may play a part, although a secondary part in the onset and prevalence of the disease."

It sounds as though she had her back to the wall defending the indefensible, but it was largely the scientific evidence of Fish's experiments that finally demolished her theories. It was an attack which aimed at her competence as a scientist, and worse, made by a clinician, one of a tribe that she always accused of seeing the problem in a superficial way. However Fish was carrying out this research in the physiology department of University College, London, the head of which was the highly respected Professor (later Sir) Charles Lovatt Evans, who was to become a staunch supporter and friend of Fish.

It seems probable that Mrs. Mellanby's assumption that calcified tissues in teeth are subject to metabolic changes after their formation, rested on the belief that tooth tissues behave like bone. As Edward Mellanby had demonstrated, the bone in rickets did respond well to a diet in which ingredients such as those found in meat, milk, and cod liver oil were present. So teeth should respond in the same way.

But tooth tissue is not bone, and does not metabolise like bone, as John Hunter had demonstrated over a hundred years earlier. In Fish's book, "An Experimental Investigation of Enamel, Dentine and the Dental Pulp" which appeared in 1933, he quotes an extract from John Hunter's 1778, "The Natural History of the Human Teeth" where Hunter describes some of his studies of growth using red madder as a bone marker:

"Take a young animal, viz., a pig, and feed it with madder for three or four weeks; then kill the animal, and upon examination you will find the following appearance: first, if this animal had some parts of its teeth formed before the feeding with madder those parts will be known by their remaining of this natural colour; but such parts as were formed while the animal was taking the madder will be found of a red colour. This shows that it is only those parts that were forming while the animal was taking the madder that are dyed; for what were already formed will not be found in the least tinged. "... it would seem that the teeth are without absorbents, as well as other vessels... This shows that the growth of the teeth is very different from that of other bones."

While Mrs. Mellanby may not have been familiar with this part of Hunter's work, Fish certainly was. He possessed a thorough knowledge of the history of dental research, and it was the old debate about the vitality of enamel which seems to have attracted him to look at the metabolism of the dental tissues. As Fish writes, "The problem has been whether enamel was alive or not, and most investigators have expressed opinions which have earned for them the description of "vitalists" (Mummery, Boedecker) or" "non-vitalists" (Hopewell Smith)..... it has been generally assumed that the presence of organic matter in enamel must indicate that the tissue is alive. It has not been realised that non-vital organic matter of a keratinous nature might exist in a non-vital enamel, while the very presence of organic matter in enamel at all was often denied by the "non-vitalists". A further consideration that Fish talked about later in life, was that as both a dental and a medical student, he wondered why he could put infected filling material into a cavity in living (sensitive) dentine, whereas the slightest infection introduced on a foreign body into bone caused an abscess. When a student he had asked the question of one of the Honorary Dental Surgeons and was told to get on with his work and not ask questions. "It was Harold Doran - now gone to God."

Fish set out to clarify the matter, taking the premise that the presence of a free fluid pathway was essential to tissue vitality. It was obvious that blood did not circulate in dentine and enamel, but nutrients could be carried by a lymph supply providing there was some permeability in the dental tissues. He designed experiments to assess the permeability of enamel and dentine, first in dogs and then in human teeth.

He looked at 132 teeth from 17 dogs, ages ranging from 9 months to 9 years. There must have been many stray dogs available at that time, and it is unlikely that the anti-vivisection movement, although very active through such organisations as the Canine Defence League, might have heard about his work at UCL or the Hampton Hale laboratory. Too many people, especially in London, lived on the bread-line to be very concerned about animal welfare, and the notion of 'animal rights' would have seemed ludicrous to many.

Fish's experiments on dogs, which were carried out under general anaesthesia, were divided into two groups in order to study, first the permeability of enamel from the dentine side, and then from the oral surface into the enamel.

In the first group a hole was drilled into the pulp and a crumb of methyl blue inserted into the hole for diffusion from the pulp through the dentine to the enamel. In the second group a dome shaped cap full of solid methyl blue powder was fixed over the enamel.

The teeth were extracted and ground sections made using a modification of a machine devised by G.V.Black. In the investigations of the structure of enamel, Fish had the help of a physicist, Dr. J. Thewlis at the National Physical Laboratory, Thewlis used the new X-ray diffraction techniques to examine the crystallographic structure of the enamel. Before 1915 it was known that the wavelength of X-rays is of the same order of magnitude as the inter-atomic distances, and Sir William Bragg with his son, devised the first X-ray spectrometer, for which they were given the Nobel prize for physics in 1925. This is the technique used thirty years later to define the structure of DNA.

Thewlis's findings were very important to the debate about the significance of faults in tooth structure found on histological examination. Margaret Murray, a junior colleague of Mrs. Mellanby's at Bedford College for Women, had recorded that she found quantitative chemical differences associated with the histological faults in enamel, a finding that would have provided some support for the Mellanby theory.

However Thewlis's crystallographic analysis did not show any difference in the region of these faults.

In the perfusion experiments on young dogs the dye was found to penetrate from the dentine to the oral surface of the enamel, and in transverse sections it was seen that the dye traversed the prism sheaths. Fish concluded that this showed free fluid flow across enamel from dentine to oral surface. With age the extent of dye penetration reduced showing that the organic material becomes less permeable. Fish argued that as the enamel in young dogs was fully calcified because the ameloblasts had already died, and calcification cannot continue in the absence of cells, this decreasing permeability was due to increasing keratinisation of the organic material with age. Also when the enamel was decalcified the organic residue was insoluble.

Dye placed on the oral surface of the enamel of young dogs entered the enamel, but with age this penetration reduced to zero in the old dogs.

From his findings where Fish had placed dye in the pulps of hundreds of extracted human teeth he concluded, "Human enamel has never in a single instance shown a degree of permeability in any way comparable to that of dog's enamel." In this respect he found that monkeys' teeth were similar to humans'.

He proceeded to ask the question: is dentine irrigated by free tissue fluid? If substances introduced into the general circulation could be detected later in the dentine that would seem to indicate free tissue fluid in the dentine. For this enquiry Fish used cats and dogs into which trypan blue was injected twice a week for two or three weeks.

The dye was found in the space between Tomes fibrils and the wall of the dentinal tubule, and Fish observed," whole tubular systems were normally in fluid communication with the pulp." He confirmed this finding by injecting India ink directly into the pulps of dog and monkey teeth. The space between fibrils and dentinal tubule walls was filled with dye. In extracted human teeth the tubules were not completely patent indicating that free circulation had been impaired. Secondary dentine blocked the way.

Fish went on to enquire what metabolic changes might take place in dentine. He writes, "When it was found that free tissue fluid was present in the dentine it seemed possible that metabolic changes might be found to occur in the tissue. The most convenient method of investigating this possibility was to carry out a series of calcium estimations upon specimens of dentine taken from teeth under circumstances which might be expected to modify their calcium content."

With the help of a famous nutritionist, Professor Drummond of University College, estimations of calcium content were carried out on normal adult human teeth, cat teeth before and after parathyroidectomy, pregnant dogs on a calcium deficient diet, dogs of various ages with increasing doses of calciferol (Vitamin D) added to the diet until the dose was so high (400,000 units of Vitamin D) that the dogs became comatose and died, and finally two dogs that as Fish describes them, were "not in normal health."

Fish summarised the results as follows:

"The calcium content of the unaffected dentine of teeth which have become carious is normal. It has not been found possible to modify the calcium content of the dentine by either in parathyroidectomy, calcium deficient diet, pregnancy or feeding on therapeutic or excessive doses of Vitamin D; nor did two dogs with extreme natural softening of the bones show any loss of calcium from the dentine.

It appears, therefore, that the calcium content of the dentine is extremely stable, that slight physiological additions may be made to it , but that there is no evidence as yet of any definite loss of calcium from the dentine under any circumstances."

He did add a rider to the effect that "Calcium salts are sometimes added to the dentine in response to local injury, in the form of a translucent zone."

This work, which clarified the nature of the response of the dental pulp to injury, was carried out at the Hale Laboratory and the physiology department of University College London, and in 1933 Fish was awarded a D.Sc. by that college. His experiments had extended over eight years, 235 teeth had been operated on, and 20,000 serial sections prepared. When in 1932 the research appeared in book form, with eight colour plates and fifty-one black and white illustrations, letters of congratulations poured in from all over the world. Requests to be able to use some of the illustrations came from workers in the field; the "colour drawings and plates are some of the most beautiful it has ever been my pleasure to study.." was a typical comment on the illustrations. They were drawn by a Miss Eleanor Dale to whom Fish acknowledges his debt. The design of the book was so innovative that the Secretary of the BDA wrote to Fish, "why nobody ever realised that there was a method of overcoming the annoyance one encounters in referring to plates and text at the same time I cannot conceive, but your publishers certainly have succeeded."

A review in the British Medical Journal described the research as "work of outstanding merit." The Journal of Pathology and Bacteriology was even more laudatory. "Dr. Fish has added an illuminating chapter to the general pathology of the defence of the body against injuries which might well be used for the instruction of medical as well as dental students."

In the acknowledgements, Fish also expresses his thanks for financial support from the Dental Board and from the MRC. Despite increasing antagonism from the Mellanbys, Fish sent a copy of his book to May Mellanby, and received a very courteous reply thanking him for "a copy of your wonderful book. What energy you have. How I wish I could express myself as easily as you do. Many congratulations."

In 1932 Fish presented a paper on the 'Aetiology of Dental Caries', which was reported in the BMJ in October of that year. After Fish had described the various types of caries, e.g. interstitial, cervical, fissure, and recurrent, members of the audience expressed an assortment of divergent views on the subject. Fish had insisted that the cause of caries was 'saprophytic', that is, produced by the oral flora. Mrs. Mellanby stated that "the structure of the tooth was one of the highest importance", and Dr.I.H.MacLean, the bacteriologist at St. Mary's Hospital, who was to work closely with Fish, believed the primary cause was an enamel fault. The Royal Dental Hospital veterans, J.G.Turner and Colyer agreed that the stagnation of fermentable carbohydrate was "the one factor beyond doubt", while Warwick James criticised the view that caries could be explained by reference to tooth structure, and emphasised the importance of B. acidophilus. Inevitably Broderick maintained that "an imbalance in the metabolic equation" was the problem.

In 1933 the Royal College of Surgeons appointed Fish the John Tomes Prizeman, a singularly appropriate award, for Fish's histological work followed closely in Tomes' footsteps. In the same year Fish was also awarded the first Howard Mummery Prize.

The whole dental profession was behind Fish. In a review paper 'Is Enamel a Vital Tissue' in the magazine 'Public Health' in 1933, Jeffery Fletcher, a school dental officer wrote, "we must continue to look on enamel, with Dr.E.W.Fish, as an inert substance." All the evidence was contrary to Mrs. Mellanby's contentions, that there is a relationship between tooth structure and susceptibility to caries, that lack of calcium and phosphorus is a cause of caries, and that a diet rich in these substances even after the eruption of teeth affects resistance to caries.

Her views, backed as they were by the MRC continued to be accepted by the medical profession, who generally refused to accept Sim Wallace's recommendations about diet, that is until Sir Arthur MacNalty, then Chief Medical Officer to the Ministry of Health, declared clearly that "a smaller consumption of bread, biscuits, sugar and sweets is the best means of the prevention of caries." On his retirement MacNalty became the editor-in-chief of the official medical history of the Second World War.

However, in the Mellanby camp Fish continued to be an unpopular man. Antagonism must have started early in the research, because there is a letter from Margaret Murray dated March 1928 from Bedford College, which criticises Fish because, "he assumes no-one (before him) knows or has examined ... methyl blue....Publishes with too little evidence." These were accusations that Mrs. Mellanby was also to make, and increasing rancour between the parties is shown in a letter from Dr. Thewlis at the National Physical Laboratory to Mrs. Mellanby, which begins, "The idea of your stealing E.W.F's work is preposterous." It seems that Fish had complained that Mrs. Mellanby had looked at the X-ray diffraction photographs of enamel that Thewlis had produced for Fish. This was probably an innocent act; perhaps Thewlis was showing Mrs. Mellanby results of which he was proud, but it does demonstrate Fish's sensitivity about his work which he considered completely original, a tendency in research which is not uncommon, especially when the researcher feels that the confidentiality of his or her ongoing findings is threatened.

Many people came to Mrs. Mellanby for her opinion about their work. She gave of her time and special knowledge unstintingly, her criticism was detailed and without compromise. Occasionally she would ask her husband's opinion, especially where the research worker sought a grant from the MRC. She seems to have reserved much time and forensic energy for an analysis of Fish's work, and wrote lengthy reports on his work. Her file on Fish is comprehensive. She collected reprints of all his articles, even including those on denture construction, and sometimes tried to recruit to her side the support of other dental scientists, including that of H.H. Stones, Fish's contemporary in Manchester.

Her marginal comments are revealing of something more than a simple difference of opinion; "utter nonsense", "not intelligible", "a specious argument." Like her colleague, Margaret Murray, she accused him of not acknowledging the work of his predecessors, and of presenting all his ideas as original. In the main her criticisms were not justified, except perhaps in her comment on a crucial statement in Fish's long article on periodontal disease. In this Fish argued that in the production of gingivitis, neither chemical nor bacterial irritation could reach gingival connective tissue because the gingival epithelium is at first completely intact over the patches of sub-epithelial round cell infiltration, therefore the cause of this inflammatory response must be mechanical. Harsh particles of food injured the fragile (because insufficiently keratinised) gingivae. She comments that, "where nutritive material can go, presumably irritants can go,"

But her feelings were clearly revealed in a letter she wrote in 1938 to Professor J.A.Ryle, Director of the recently formed Institute of Social Medicine in Oxford, who had asked her opinion of current dental research. "I want to speak to you as a friend," Lady Mellanby wrote. She proceeded to comment on research at various dental institutions. UCH Dental School was "hopeless", and that at the Royal Dental Hospital , "worse than UCH". In giving her opinion of people in dental research she praised Dr.J.D. King , who had MRC support and was later to become its dental director. He was, although rather rough, she thought reliable, as was a young gentleman at Guy's, a Cambridge man, one Martin Rushton, who was to become a highly respected professor of Oral Medicine, and Dean of the Faculty of Dental Science at the Royal College of Surgeons. Of Fish she wrote, "I think him a dishonest research worker, but a very clever (too clever) man; who has, I believe, hindered honest dental research…I think EWF too keen on social advancement on past research." A wonderfully revealing expression of how the

Mellanbys, upper middle-class Cambridge graduates and members of the scientific elite, regarded this red-brick university educated son of the manse.

There are also remarks about Fish personally, especially his boasting of how much he was earning in private practice. No doubt his earnings were greater than that of both Mellanby's together. May Mellanby concluded her comments with, "He is just a social climber. (He wanted to get FRS and said Sir Walter would have seen to this, but not EM, hence....!!)."

The dental profession's opinion of May Mellanby reciprocated her view of the profession. In later years she complained that their treatment of her when invited to lecture was shabby; no one met her at railway stations, payment of her fee was delayed, and altogether she felt, entirely because she was a woman. Their behaviour did the profession no credit, but she could not accept that her theories were wrong. A more professional view was expressed by Colyer, who regarded her as a harmful intruder into matters over which she had little competence. Colyer had scathing opinions about many of his contemporaries. He regarded Bradlaw with contempt, no doubt because of the latter's attack on the power of the part-time Honoraries, and he was reluctant to praise Fish, although he respected his sharp brain.

The minutes of the Royal Society are available for inspection, but delicate matters, such as the fortunes of an application are kept secret. Fish's name is on the files of the Society, therefore one must conclude that his name was put forward for election to a Fellowship, by whom is not recorded, but nothing came of it. To be elected to a Fellowship of the Royal Society is the ultimate British scientific accolade. According to the statute of the Society at that time, it was awarded to "Men (women were not recognised until the Second World War) distinguished in the scientific or educational service of the State, or by their services to science and its application". The list of Fellows reads like a pantheon of scientific deities, including Einstein and Freud, and Nobel Laureates in all scientific fields. In 1937, Sir W.H. Bragg was President, William Trotter, Surgeon to the king, and Nobel Laureate, Professor James Chadwick, were on the main committee. A nominee for fellowship had to be proposed and recommended by a certificate signed by six Fellows, and his case put for consideration to a selection committee. In Fish's case this would have been the 'Animal Physiology and Medicine' Board, on which sat eight eminent scientists, including Edward Mellanby.

It is likely that the personal animosity between Fish and the Mellanbys represented an important factor in the rejection of Fish's candidature, but this was not necessarily the only consideration. Both academic status and value of research were considered. Many candidates were Fellows of Oxford or Cambridge colleges, or heads of important institutes In 1937 the twenty-one new Fellows included D.R.Pye, Director of Scientific Research at the Air Ministry, and the eminent pathologist, A.N.Drury, Fellow of Trinity College. Fish held no formal academic appointment, and never had. His research activity was part-time, and no doubt in the eyes of many (as he himself was to declare) was subordinate to his clinical practice. It is also possible that his work on the minutiae of dental physiology was seen as of minor importance, as were all matters dental at that time. Indeed no Fellowship had been given for research in dentistry since John and Charles Tomes in the nineteenth century. Taking his aspirations in the context of the time, it may have been premature of Fish's nominees to have attempted an exercise that could fail. Having said that, if one looks at the originality of his thinking, in which he brought science to the practice of dentistry, his contribution is certainly worthy of a Fellowship of that hallowed Society. Alas, dentistry was, as it still is in the eyes of many, a small and not too important aspect of medicine. Nevertheless the resolution and outcome of the Mellanby dispute demonstrated the calibre of dental research, and represented a positive step in furthering the reputation of the profession. In some areas the hegemony of the medical profession did nor reign supreme, and the authority of the dental profession had to be acknowledged.

The importance of Fish's contribution continued to be acknowledged abroad; in 1938 the Australian Dental Association made him an honorary member, the Netherlands bestowed the same honour in 1938, and Sweden in 1950. The BDA which had been rather tardy in its acceptance of Fish's work, gave him honorary membership in 1951, the Royal Society of Medicine in 1955, and finally the American Academy of Dentistry in 1957. At last the American profession made a public acknowledgement that some aspect of British dentistry was worthy of praise.

In February 1937 Fish asked the MRC for funds for a research secretary as he was "engaged in clinical practice and gives two days of his time each week to research work." Fish also asked for a grant increase of £40 " to enable me to engage a laboratory boy and so free Pereira (his technician who was later to do medicine) from some of the less technical tasks."

It is hardly surprising in the personal climate of that time, that at a meeting of the MRC, Dental Diseases Committee in July 1937, it was decided that Fish's MRC grant be reduced. The reason given was rather curious, " in view of the withdrawal of Dr. MacGregor, Dr. Bradlaw and Professor Stone, ... but Dr. Fish should know of our decision and given an opportunity of putting his case before the committee." Did this mean that Fish's friends and colleagues were abandoning him, or much more likely that they did not want to be party to this reduction in financial support? But Fish was not without supporters on important committees, for the report continues," ... Ballard, the new member of the Dental Board representing the 1921 men , who has fallen under the spell of Fish" ... "agrees with a reduction of £100 only when Fish goes to St. Mary's".

The dispute must have created an unhappy atmosphere for all in any way involved, and in June 1939 Margaret Murray wrote to Edward Mellanby to say that she was thinking of resigning from the MRC Advisory Committee because she was unhappy about the argument between dental clinicians and scientific workers.

If the Mellanbys thought that they could deal with Fish as they had with Weaver, they were very much mistaken. Fish was not a government servant, indeed he was nobody's servant, and perfectly capable of financing his own research if need be. Although he always contended that he was a clinician with research as a hobby, the two activities were intimately connected, both technically and financially. By 1939 with most of his research activity behind him, Fish had made himself completely independent, and ready to engage in dental politics. He had already made his mark in the Federation Dentaire Internationale, where national prestige weighed heavily in decision making.

Fish must have met May Mellanby at conferences, as well as her husband, if only at the offices of the MRC when he applied for grants or went to made progress reports on his work. No doubt the conventions of polite behaviour concealed any professional antagonism, and despite all the clinical and scientific evidence that was mounted against Mrs. (now Lady) Mellanby's ideas, the row persisted, especially given Edward Mellanby's support for his wife. In 1938 Sir Norman Bennett, who had helped steer the 1921 Dentists Act through parliament, and had been President of the BDA in 1930, wrote, "I suppose that the nutrition experts seem to be too much inclined to ignore completely the physical structure of food-stuffs." And in the Lancet of 1942, commenting on Sir Edward Mellanby's defence of wartime measure of adulterating bread with chalk to provide calcium, and his assertion that without the additional calcium caries would be even worse, Bennett wrote that first, there is no evidence that calcium in diet makes a difference because, caries always starts on the surface of enamel, and second, there is no evidence that calcium in diet affects enamel once it is formed."

It is characteristic of Fish that he made no public criticism of Mrs. Mellanby. Later in life, his comment on this work (quoted earlier) was , "Looking at as a whole this series of experiments did make filling a tooth an intelligent and intelligible operation as far as I am concerned , and if I hadn't done it I am pretty sure that I should have switched into surgery - either general or specialized, in some other, better understood field."

The question, what is the scientific basis for the things we do to our patients?, underpinned all Fish's research, and this is no more clearly shown than in his work on Focal Infection.

Chapter 9

FOCAL INFECTION

At a joint meeting of several sections of the Royal Society of Medicine, held in 1925 to discuss the topic, 'Focal Infection as a Factor in Disease', Mr. G. A. Peake, a dental surgeon from Cheltenham, reported on an interesting case: "A retired army major of fine physique and a very good cricketer" complained of tingling and numbness of his right arm. The Wasserman test (for syphilis) was negative, he had a clean mouth, healthy gums and was free of caries. As there was no obvious cause for his symptoms Mr. Peake extracted all the major's teeth, and six months later all power returned to his arm. Years after Mr. Peake mused, "he is still grateful to me but I often wonder whether with the very slight physical signs in his mouth I was right in extracting all his teeth."

Even in 1925, the possibility of a connection between playing cricket and damage to the brachial plexus, must have been considered, especially if the major had been a right-handed fast bowler. Presumably Mr. Peake, as a Member or even Fellow of the Royal Society of Medicine, was doubly qualified like most members at that time, and therefore informed about parts of the body other than the mouth. But without an obvious causal factor, some hidden focus, and particularly a dental one, had to be considered as the likely culprit.

So many diseases were of mysterious origin, especially those that were chronic in nature: arthritis, sciatica, peripheral neuritis, headaches, migraine, asthma, pernicious anaemia, gastric ulcers, kidney disease were attributed to the presence of some distant focus. "Acute pancreatitis may follow oral sepsis, possibly by way of an ascending infection from the bowel.....septicaemia and malignant carditis might also be caused," was the sober conclusion of one physician.

At the same meeting other anecdotes of a similar nature were related, and some firmly held opinions implicated disease in various parts of the body as foci of infection. In particular the tonsils, adenoids, sinuses, teeth and gums, boils, septic gall bladders, and a variety of gastro-intestinal lesions were named as foci from where toxins were conveyed by the blood. Even mental diseases might be caused by such foci. A Dr. T.C.Graves described a case of mental disorder in this way. " Photographs show depressed facial appearance of a young married woman the subject of melancholia." Three carious teeth and a buried root were removed, and some 'uterine endocervicitis' was treated. "A photograph taken three weeks later shows an improved facial appearance and... a fortnight later a still happier facial aspect." Perhaps constant and low-grade discomfort from her several maladies had made the young lady miserable, and the removal of the causes had improved her mood, but no explanation of that sort seems to have been considered; the melancholia was deemed to be the direct result of toxins from these septic foci somehow affecting the nervous system.

At an earlier meeting of the RSM in 1924, no less a person than the highly respected bacteriologist and government advisor, Sir Kenneth Goadby, winner of the John Tomes Prize of 1903, had expressed the view that, "The mouth as a focus of infection is now regarded as the source of a large number of the diseases from which modern civilization suffers."

In his introductory lecture to the 1925 meeting, Professor G.R. Murray provided a comprehensive review of scientific opinion at that time. He said, "During recent years much attention has been drawn to the subject selected for discussion today, and we have learned how important a part focal sepsis may play in the causation of disease, and in the progress of a malady already present...a malady may be initiated or its course affected by a local infection in several different ways.

Professor Murray went on to detail the various pathways involved in the slow and continuous seepage of toxins into the bloodstream. This notion of toxic seepage is at the heart of the concept of focal infection. The systematic study of those inborn defences against infection that constitute the immune system, was to be some time in the future; its only expression at that time lay in the words, "local resistance" and "arrested by the nearest lymph gland."

These views clearly revealed the limitations of medical knowledge at that time. They also reflect the prevalence of uncontrolled and debilitating diseases which impair the resistance of the patient to the spread of bacteria and toxins. But a diagnosis had to be made, treatment was expected, this was the age of science, the doctor must avoid a show of ignorance, and action was imperative. When it came to it, tonsils, adenoids, appendices and teeth were expendable, so they had to go. And they did. The removal of tonsils and adenoids had by then become routine, and even as late as the early part of the twentieth century, often performed on the kitchen table without anaesthesia.

At a meeting of the Odontological Section of the RSM held in January 1920, Mr. F. St. J. Steadman read a paper on Dental Sepsis in Children, in which the consequences of sepsis in the mouth spilling into the bloodstream were spelled out. Apart from gastro-intestinal upset, wasting, fretfulness and night terrors, Mr. Steadman described septicaemia, endocarditiis and the potential of affected lymph glands to become tubercular. His prescription was the extraction of all infected teeth and their antagonists, which if left in would become tender and lead to unilateral mastication. Furthermore, by such extractions, he explained, "the area of mastication was increased." His final advice was that, "If extensive extraction has to be done, the operation should be completed at one time under a general anaesthetic such as ethyl chloride." This advice at a time when death from chloroform and ethyl chloride anaesthesia was tragically common, especially among children. Visits to the dentist were always feared, and understandably so.

Even until comparatively recently complete tooth extractions were ordered prior to major surgery, often reducing the patient to complete psychological despair as well as physical debility.

Despite the conviction of many at the meeting of the almost universal importance of focal infection there were more cautious voices. A Mr. Thomson, when talking about arthritis expressed the opinion, "Though chronic disease of the teeth, tonsils, urinary tract, and other organs is almost universally common, only a small proportion of cases develop multiple arthritis."

One of the most respected dental surgeons present at the 1925 meeting was F.W.Broderick, described by the editor of the BDJ, as a man of "compelling personality and incomprehensible theories". He was the author of a monumental text, 'The Principles of Dental Medicine', in which he proposed the theory that caries and pyorrhoea were opposite and distinct diseases, both being the result of general rather than local causes but dependent on opposite and antagonistic states of the system, such as variation in the acidity or alkalinity of an individual's metabolism. A review of Broderick's work in the BDJ states caustically, "Though it would be incorrect and even unfair to speak of Mr. Broderick as a voice crying in the wilderness, yet as he would be the first to admit, his views are still in a pioneer stage..." After Broderick's protest, the BDJ apologised with the usual rider, "if we have misrepresented Mr. Broderick's view". His obituary was kinder, "by ascribing the causes of dental disease to general conditions he started a train of thought which may bear great fruit."

But twenty years earlier, when Broderick dealt with matters dental his views were listened to with attention, in particular his view that chronic sepsis lay in a "lack of defensive power of the body."

At the meeting he said, "The most notable thing from the point of view of the practising dentist, especially one who studies any number of radiographs, is the extraordinary number of patients who show signs of periapical absorption with presumably no symptoms of general infection, persons who are, notwithstanding this condition, in perfect health. On the other hand one cannot fail to be struck by the enormous improvement that does occasionally take place on the removal of infected teeth in certain cases referred to us by medical practitioners. Further it is not necessarily in those cases in which the sepsis would seem to be greatest that symptoms of general involvement always show themselves."

He then went on to speak specifically about dental sepsis. "A tooth in which the pulp has been destroyed, and which contains an infected pulp chamber, is a very difficult problem from the point of view of body defence, since it is impossible , however well the blood may be circumstanced to overcome that infection. The micro-organisms entrenched within the tooth are able to draw their sustenance by way of the lymphatics in the periodontal membrane, though the root tissue, while they themselves remain there inviolable and protected from the blood stream."

"Now it happens that the very presence of a granuloma, recognised by an area of rarefaction at this spot, is as a rule sufficient, in the minds of most men, to condemn the teeth, as being in itself proof of infection, whereas in reality it shows the reaction of the body to the infection, and in many cases a very satisfactory reaction."

It is more than likely that Fish attended this meeting. A year earlier he had given a lecture to the British Society of Dental Surgeons on the influence of oral sepsis, and Broderick's statement could well be read as an introduction to Fish's own research.

By the beginning of the twentieth century, with improvements in dental materials and techniques, dentists became more ambitious in their efforts to save teeth and avoid removable appliances. The ability to provide efficient and aesthetic crowns and bridgework became a measure of the dental art, and by 1910 root canal treatment had reached such a degree of effectiveness that , as the eminent Australian endodontist, F.J.Harty, wrote, "no self respecting dentist would extract a tooth. Every stump was retained and a porcelain or gold crown constructed. Fistulas appeared often and were treated by various methods for years on end if necessary. The connection between the fistula and the dead tooth was known but not acted upon."

The medical application of X-rays followed swiftly after its discovery in 1895 by the German physicist Wilhelm Rontgen, and in fact amongst the first x-ray photographs that he produced was one of the bones of his wife's hand. Only two days after the publication of Rontgen's paper a Scottish surgeon used x-rays to observe the withdrawal of a needle from an unfortunate seamstresses' hand, and the application of x-rays for the examination of the dentition (the intra-oral skiagrams as they were then called) was not delayed. As well as the alveolar bone destruction of pyorrhoea the skiagrams revealed a sorry tale of inadequate root treatment and apical pathology, and the extraction of such teeth often revealed large granulomatous masses attached to the roots. Not surprisingly the sight of such lesions caused great alarm to both dentist and patient. Apprehension about the hazard of diseased teeth was compounded by the regular finding of bacteria around the apex of teeth after extraction.

One major handicap to successful root canal treatment was ineffective sterilisation, only chemical disinfectants were used, and the average dental surgery with its fabric covered chair, foot engine and insanitary spittoon, provided excellent breeding conditions for bacteria. It is little wonder that in 1911 the British physician, William Hunter, in an article in The Lancet, attacked 'American dentistry', which he blamed for numerous diseases of unknown origin, and he reported cases of recovery from illness following tooth extraction. In 1918 the American physician, F. Billings, coined the term, 'focal infection'. Hunter's condemnation started a vigorous reaction to tooth conservation, and in particular to root canal treatment. Could the whole exercise of root canal treatment be a hazard to health, and if it was, could it ever be justified? As a report of the Scientific Committee of the International Dental Federation in 1928 stated, " a diagnosis of apical infection is to many doctors and to some dentists the equivalent of a sentence of death on the affected teeth which allows of no reprieve."

Both non-vital and healthy teeth were removed wherever some disease of obscure origin was diagnosed. This was especially the case in Britain, where wholesale extraction began. It was less so on the Continent, perhaps because the Germans, French and other Europeans put a higher value on their teeth. When in the 'thirties many Europeans fleeing the Nazis arrived in

Britain, two of their important needs were central heating and a dentist who didn't extract teeth. Fortunately for them there were many such dentists among their number.

In 1923 Fish was invited to give the paper referred to above, to the British Society of Dental Surgeons (also known as Colyer's Society). Colyer thought that the only portal to the Dental Register was the LDS diploma and he was vigorously opposed to the inclusion of '1921 men' in the Dental Register, and once this had happened his Society was disbanded. Originally Fish had been invited to talk on 'Some difficulties in dental practice', but as someone else had given an excellent paper on that subject, Fish chose to speak on, 'The Influence of the Occurrence of General Absorption on the Treatment of Oral Sepsis'. In that paper he said, "It is generally accepted that oral sepsis is very often the cause of a large group of diseases from tonsillitis and gastritis to rheumatism, deranged action of the heart and chronic mania; but this statement does not go unchallenged." He went on to cite the views of F.W.Broderick, one of which was that pyorrhoea "is the result of seruminal calculus deposited below the gum margin from saliva in which lime salts are present." At the end of the paper Fish presented a suggested 'case sheet' for dentists to follow in taking a history and examining the patient, using as an example a patient with gout and dental abscesses. He concluded, "the coincidence between the first attack of gout and the commencement of oral sepsis in point of time suggests a causal relationship with lowering of the resistance as the determining factor of each attack." Almost half a century later, in 1971, when Fish was reviewing and ordering his work for his friend and former colleague, H.M. Pickard, his acid comment on this paper was, "What cheek!"

In 1925 and now the possessor of an MD, Fish wrote an article, 'The Mouth as a Focus of Infection', for the 'Royal Dental Hospital Reports'. In this, his first article after his appointment at RDH, he comments on the size of the problem, "it is unnecessary to emphasize the almost universal incidence of oral sepsis amongst the adult population of civilized countries," and he goes on to consider a problem that every dentist faced, the difficulty of deciding on the merits of removing all apparent sources of oral sepsis against the trauma of multiple extractions and the difficulty of denture wearing. He writes, "Our decision must depend upon the extent to which toxins are being absorbed with consequent impairment of the patient's health. How do we determine this?

"Toxaemia is the resultant of two opposing factors - the virulence of the bacterial attack and the efficiency of the patient's defences. The widespread presence of pus in adult mouths shows that the tissues are destroyed locally by the infection. In most cases, however, a barrier is set up round the site of infection which is sufficient to localise the invasion completely. If however the barrier should prove inefficient and septic absorption set in, the patient then presents a clinical picture which it is most important to recognize, for upon its recognition will depend our decision as to whether the teeth must be extracted or not."

Fish describes the objective signs of toxaemia, such as a reduction of red cells and haemoglobin, or a leucopenia, but adds, "It must be admitted.... these pathological investigations are not of very great help to the clinician."

The article demonstrates the difficulty of relating a specific local lesion to the general condition of the patient, and Fish expresses his caution when he writes, " it might be urged that a mild attack of sciatica, for instance, is not sufficient justification for the extraction of a number of teeth" and in addressing considerations of age, he concludes, "Later in life - after the 60th year has been passed - it is very questionable whether even extraction of all the teeth will eradicate the sepsis from the maxilla ... in old age the discomfort, annoyance and shock caused by the operation of extraction and the subsequent insertion of dentures is a far greater trial than most of the illnesses the original sepsis might lead to, or indeed than death itself."

It is a pity that more doctors and dentists of the time did not possess such a sense of proportion, or understanding of the trauma of loss of teeth. But at that time Fish's view of focal infection was essentially the same as that of Professor Murray, and in his paper he cites a case of a young woman with a history of severe neurasthesia which he links with apical infection. Even the fact that disease in other parts of the body persisted after total extractions did not modify the view taken by most doctors and dentists of focal infection.

This view is dramatically highlighted in a story that Fish tells about a child patient that some years later, Sir William Wilcox, the Home Office pathologist in the Crippen trial, asked him to see. "One day Wilcox asked me to see a child who had a rheumatic (non-infective) endocarditis. The child had a chronic but active gingivitis and some caries. The (nursing) Sister received me in frigid silence and I saw the child. In order to prevent a bacterial shower which (this was before penicillin) might have been fatal, I prescribed a soft diet, no hard food of any kind, no toothbrush - just gentle lavage of teeth and gums with $H_2 O_2$. The Sister, to whom I explained the reason for this novel treatment, suddenly became charming and brightened up. She said that her concern had been that I would want to extract the teeth after which operation all her previous children had died."

Fish cites two obvious dental examples of "perfect foci of infection", as he described them, "the ulcer in the pyorrhetic pocket of a loose tooth" which may give rise to a bacteriaemia during eating or dental treatment, especially in extraction, and the apical granuloma of a firmly implanted tooth.

The spread of bacteria and toxins from the pyorrhoea pocket did not appear to present much mystery, but many uncertainties surrounded apical infection. Was an apical radiolucency seen on x-ray, or even the presence of a granuloma always a focus of infection; was a dead or gangrenous pulp always a danger to general health; indeed one of Fish's early experiments in this field was founded on his questioning the finding of bacterial contamination of the tooth root after extraction. He suspected that where some periodontal disease was present, the compression and twisting movements of extraction would produce a bacteraemia which could contaminate the more apical surfaces of the root. To obviate this process of contamination he cauterised inflamed gingival tissue plus any periodontal pocket and infected root surface prior to extraction. His suspicion was found to be correct for where the root was healthy no bacteria were found.

But this evidence was no defence against the attacks on root canal treatment. Much more needed to be done, and following the report of the FDI's Scientific Commissions, Fish wrote a letter to the BDJ saying, "The fact that so many authorities condemn the practice of treating root canals as dangerous to the health of the patient renders it incumbent upon those who follow this practice to demonstrate to the entire satisfaction of the medical and dental professions that such treatment can result in a perfectly healthy condition of the periapical tissues. To enable them to do this the International Dental Federation has decided to offer a gold medal and a substantial prize of about £200 for the most efficient root canal technique ... several of the most eminent pathologists in Europe and America will act as judges." Fish goes on to say that as x-ray examination is not sufficient the Scientific Commission "have therefore decided to adopt the biological technique devised by Dr. Gottlieb"

Gottlieb was then the President of the Scientific Commission, and dominated the field of dental histology. His technique for assessing the condition of the apical tissues after root canal treatment was as follows:

Root canal treatment was carried out on a condemned tooth, and prior to extraction the related gingiva was painted with iodine and cauterised so that no periodontal infection could be carried to the apical tissues. Under strictly controlled sterile conditions the apex of the filled tooth was cut off and implanted into the leg muscle of a rat. After a few months the rat was killed and the leg muscles sectioned with the apex *in situ*. Where the root canal had been effectively sterilised and filled the connective tissue around the apex was perfectly healthy, but where an unfilled canal or unfilled lateral canal was left containing infection the surrounding rat tissue showed leucocyte infiltration.

Gottlieb carried out this experiment with several variations, e.g. where the extracted tooth was healthy, had an apical granuloma, a gangrenous pulp, and where different forms of root canal treatment had been used. Gottlieb was able to demonstrate that where all root canals including lateral canals were sterilised and occluded no apical infection occurred and efficient root canal treatment presented no danger to the patient's general health. This investigation amounted to almost one hundred experiments, after which Gottlieb gave Fish a complete set of the slides. Their relationship was one of mutual respect, and Fish always acknowledged his debt to the older man.

Further evidence that movement of teeth could induce the spread of bacteria in the bloodstream was provided by Okell and Elliott in 1935, when they recovered oral bacteria from the median basilic vein a few minutes after tooth extraction, and then the following year by Round, Kirkpatrick and Hails, who reported finding oral bacteria in the circulation of patients with pyorrhoea after chewing hard sweets. Fish also produced evidence of this 'bacterial shower' when he found bacteria in the pulps of recently extracted teeth.

The danger of such bacterial showers in patents with heart defects had long been recognised. As Fish wrote, ".. there can be little doubt that the bacteriaemia caused by masticating hard food or by tooth extraction is a grave menace to a patient suffering from rheumatic endocarditis with vegetations on the heart valves." (He could well have included the scaling procedure as a potential cause of infective endocarditis in the vulnerable patient). The central dilemma was how to deal with the patient presenting with dental infection, either periapical or periodontal, who had a heart problem. Was treatment of the infection more or less hazardous than extraction? One such problem was Vincent's Disease, or Acute Ulcerative Gingivitis. This was more commonly known then as Trench Mouth because of its common occurrence in the appalling conditions suffered by soldiers in the First World War, and was a very common condition in young adults, seen frequently at dental schools. Some of these patients had heart disease. Any kind of manipulation, in particular extractions, would have put the patient's life in danger, and Fish used a regime devised by the Canadian, H.K.Box, who taught at Toronto University Dental School, in which gentle packing of the gingival pocket with shredded cotton wool coated with zinc oxide and oil of cloves was carried out until the infection subsided, after which careful cleaning could be performed. This technique was used until the advent of antibiotics over twenty years later.

In 1936 Fish published a paper, 'The distribution of oral streptococci in the tissues' based on research which later in life he described as, "one of the most valuable bits of research I did because it seemed to give me a clear picture of what effect oral infections could have had on the general health (frankly, very little). Whereas ten years earlier every disease from Diabetes to Pernicious Anaemia and Rheumatoid Arthritis was due to, or influenced by Oral Sepsis (… and see my infantile efforts in 1924 before I had done any research on it.- what cheek)"

In this paper, written with his colleague, Dr. I.H. MacLean, the bacteriologist at St Mary's, Fish analyses the observations made over the years from his large collection of slides from over 200 extracted teeth and periodontal tissues, and reconciles the bacteriological and histological findings. He traces the tissue response to bacterial contamination from when the Streptococcus in the bloodstream or connective tissue "is immediately surrounded by 30,000 million polynuclear leucocytes .... which treat it as food" to the stalemate situation of the necrotic nidus. He demonstrated that organisms were always confined to this necrotic nidus, and never distributed at large in the living tissue, whether in bone or in soft connective tissue. He showed that no specimen of human gum is entirely free of a round cell infiltration, and that the gingiva attached to extracted teeth is heavily infected, but that the bottom of the 'pyorrhoeic ulcer' with a massive round cell infiltration, is nevertheless sterile. Also organisms were never found in uninflamed pulps. The histological picture confirmed that where the periodontal tissues had been cauterised prior to extraction, the pulp and bone and supporting tissues were never infected. He came to the conclusion that there is "no pathological reason why every mechanically useful live tooth should not be saved." In discussing the case where extraction cannot be avoided, Fish wrote," If the extraction is delayed until the gums are perfectly pink, clean and normal in appearance.... there is no objection to using local anaesthesia, since whatever may be the case during an acute attack, it has been shown conclusively that in the absence of acute inflammation, the deep tissues are always sterile."

Fish comments about this paper that "it had a more general application and because the evidence put forward therein enabled me to give a rational answer to the physician who (some of them) still regard "focal infection" as a potent cause of all kinds of diseases. The evidence satisfied my old friend and colleague , Sir William Wilcox, who had been Home Office pathologist (The Crippen Trial!) - he no longer asked for "clearances" (Thank God!)" One can imagine the relief Fish felt when that resented burden was lifted, especially one which often condemned children to death.

In looking back on this work, Fish commented, "The idea that unless there was a necrotic nidus surrounded by polymorphs, the tissues must be free from septic organisms occurred to me in the middle of a lecture in Melbourne! - now read on."

A wonderful illustration of how frequently the obvious can be elusive, and how readily pre-occupations rise to the surface whatever else occupies the mind.

Having left RDH, Fish was working at the Meyerstein Laboratory for Dental Research at St. Mary's Hospital, and continued his collaboration with Dr. MacLean. In an article, 'The teeth as a source of focal sepsis' in the Postgraduate Medical Journal of 1940, he reiterates his earlier description of the tissue response to bacterial invasion, starting with the definition, "A focus of infection is a chronic lesion where septic organisms have secured a foothold in a necrotic nidus from which soluble toxic matter may diffuse into the adjacent living tissues and be carried thence all over the body. From such a focus those same organisms may sometimes be dislodged by relatively slight traumatic interference and propelled into the bloodstream." On the specifically dental lesion he continues, "The chronicity of the lesion depends upon the opportunity offered by the germs to maintain a footing in contact with the tissues, but protected from attack by the polymorphonuclear leucocytes. It is the unique opportunity afforded by the dental tissues for such a footing which makes them a constant source of focal infection.....The classical instance is the 'dead tooth' where there is stalemate between the organisms in the minute canals of the tooth which cannot get out because the polymorphs guard the entrance ...and although... the polymorphs can't get in, toxic products diffuse out into the tissues."

In considering the difficulties of studying the response of dental tissues to infection, he notes, "In the mouth contaminating organisms interfere with study of the effect of specific organisms, e.g. Streptococcus Viridans, but ? comparable lesions can be produced in bone."

In the experiment to study the response of bone to infection a hole was drilled into bone under sterile conditions laid down by Dr. Maclean, and a pledget of cotton wool infected with the specific organism, *Streptococcus Viridans,* was placed in the hole and the wound closed. After seven days the animal was killed and sections made of the lesion. These showed four well defined zones which Fish described as follows:

The Zone of Infection with organisms and leucocytes.

The Zone of Contamination without organisms or leucocytes but in which toxins had killed cells.

The Zone of Irritation in which osteoclasts make their first appearance

The Zone Of Stimulation in which osteoblasts are making new bone.

Similar accounts of the tissue response to infection had been given by others, but not with the clear definition of Fish's sections. He noted that the degree of bone absorption varied with the degree of irritation; that leucocytes indicate the presence of organisms; and that, "if the tissues are merely infiltrated with round cells (lymphocytes) there is only soluble toxic matter there", e.g. as in the apical granuloma.

He drew the parallel with the "pyorrhoea pocket" in which the polymorphonuclear leucocytes lie superficially while below the surface there is an extensive infiltration of round cells which demonstrates that "it is impossible to have organisms wandering around the tissues unheeded by the predatory leucocytes.".

By 1948, when Fish brought out his 'Surgical Pathology of the Mouth', medical science had moved on. As Fish could then point out, such diseases as diabetes and pernicious anaemia, formerly thought to be the results of focal infection, had scientific explanations, and could occur where patients had perfectly healthy mouths. He was able to write: "Whatever may be the actual role of oral sepsis in general disease there has, therefore, been a certain amount of overstatement."

The bitter irony in this statement is clear. Fish must have borne witness to the extraction of countless numbers of teeth without reasonable evidence of its necessity. Indeed on many occasions he must have bowed reluctantly to the insistent advice of senior medical colleagues who allowed their dogmatic belief in focal infection to override any consideration of the consequences. Alas, those consequences were all too often, not just the pain of extraction and the misery of denture-wearing but death from anaesthesia, especially in children, a not uncommon event. And not just from the anaesthetic, but also from osteomyelitis and septicaemia following infection of the extraction wound, and even from a massive cellulitis of the submandibular tissues blocking the airway. But the loss of a tooth or even all teeth was scarcely more than a trivial matter, and accidents do happen in the best regulated circumstances.

In a paper, 'The Socialist Criticism of the Medical Profession' read in 1909 to the Medico-Legal Society, Bernard Shaw, great dramatist and satirist of the medical profession, said," ...the doctor is a specially dangerous man when poor." He could have added, and when ignorant and arrogant. When in response to Sir William Wilcox's change of attitude, Fish exclaimed, "Thank God !", it must have been a cry from the very heart of his being.

In an article, 'Oral Sepsis', published in 1958, Fish presented a history of the changed view of the relationship between those foci of infection, in the mouth, tonsils, urethra and intestines, once thought to be so important in the aetiology of arthritis, fibrositis, and rheumatic disease, and summarised the responsibilities of the dental surgeon as:-

a) by leaving chronic foci of infection he is exposing the patient to risk by spreading bacteria locally, generally by bacterial shower, or into intra-vascular lesions

b) by disturbing a chronic focus in the course of treatment, he himself is taking a similar but calculated risk, and must ensure, if necessary even by the use of cautery or by antibiotic cover, or both, that the patient's health is not prejudiced.

While mysteries about disease causation and pathology persisted, the notion of focal sepsis held a strong hold, only to be attenuated slowly by scientifically based understanding of the pathogenesis of disease processes. There is no doubt that Fish's research represents a major contribution to this change.

Right: EWF with his dog Toby in his garden at Winchester

Below: Schoolboy Eric Wilfred Fish

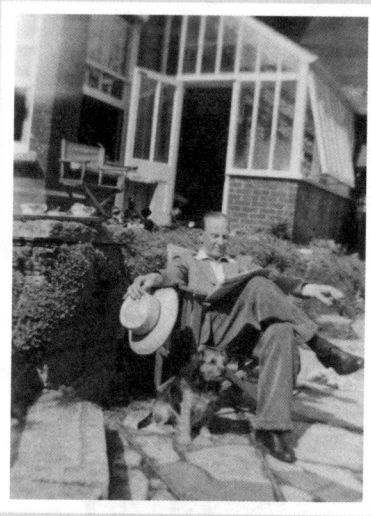

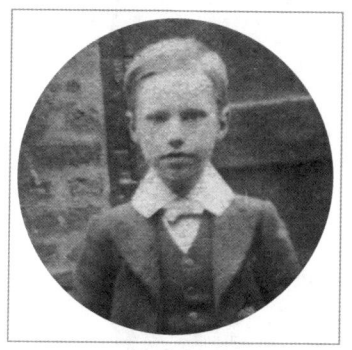

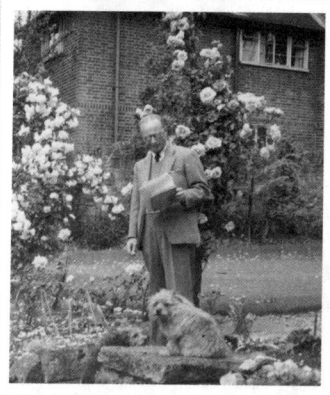

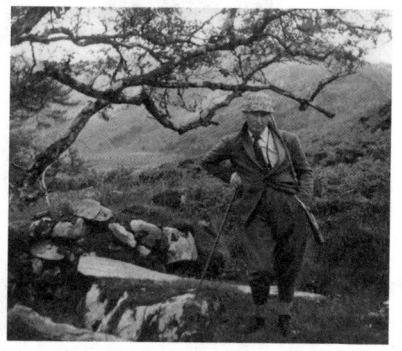

EWF always working even when in the garden with his dogs.

EWF, a first-rate shot, stalking deer at Killarney.

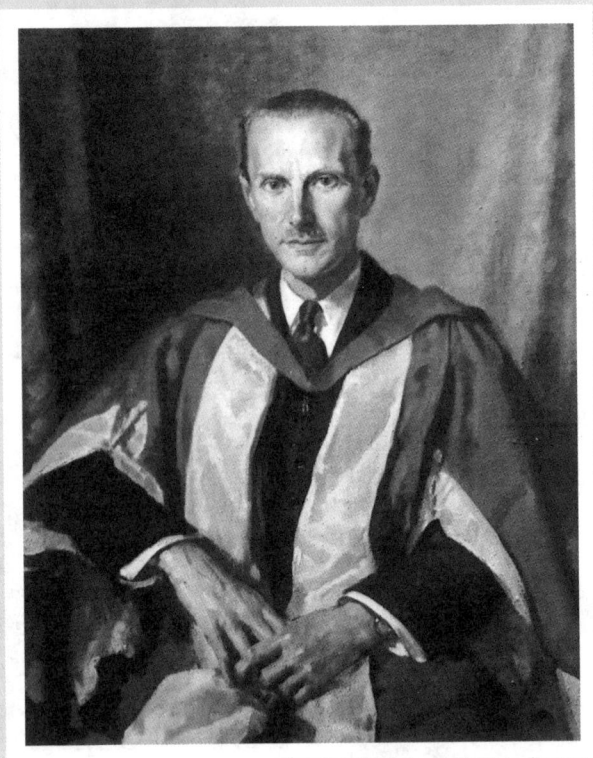

Dr. E Wilfred Fish MD DDS DSc by Francis Hodge

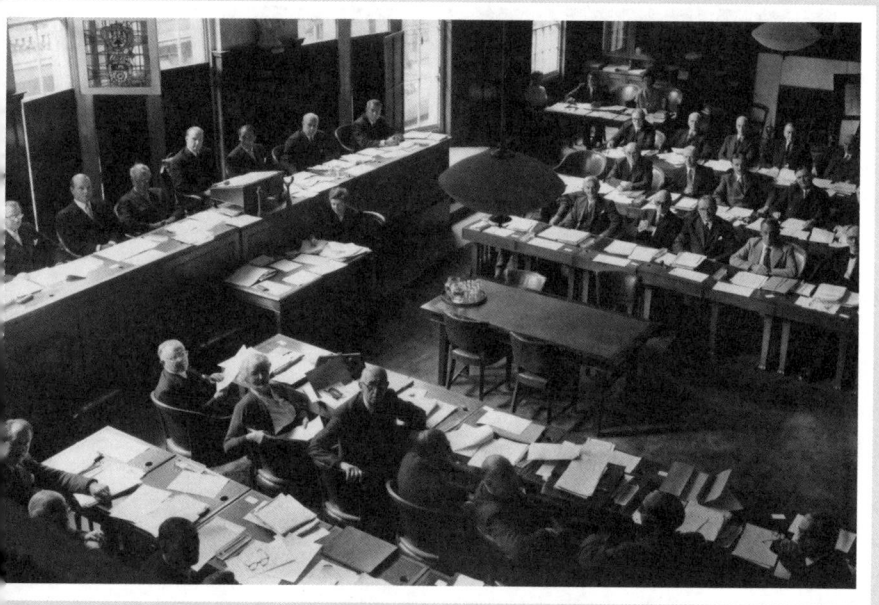

First session of the General Dental Council, July 1956
in the General Medical Council's Council Chamber, EWF in the Chair

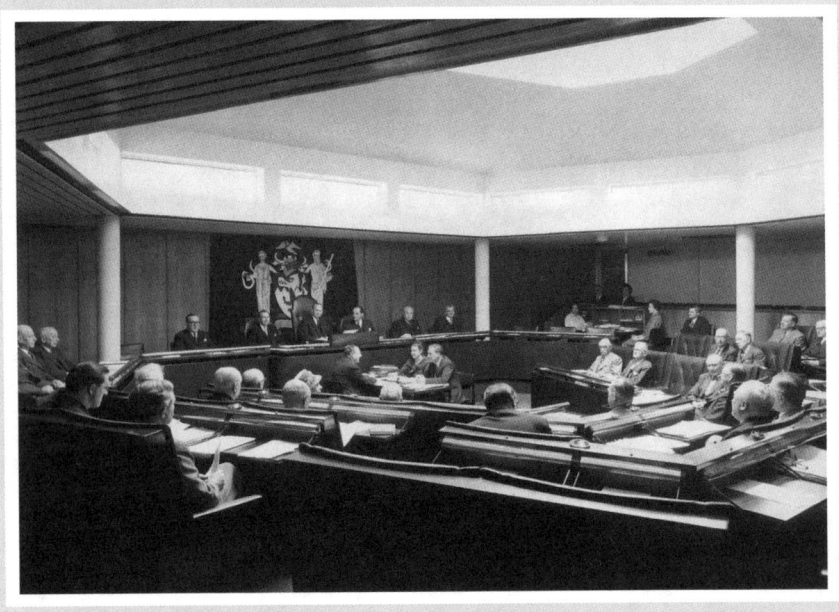

New Council Chamber, General Dental Council at 37 Wimpole Street, London W1

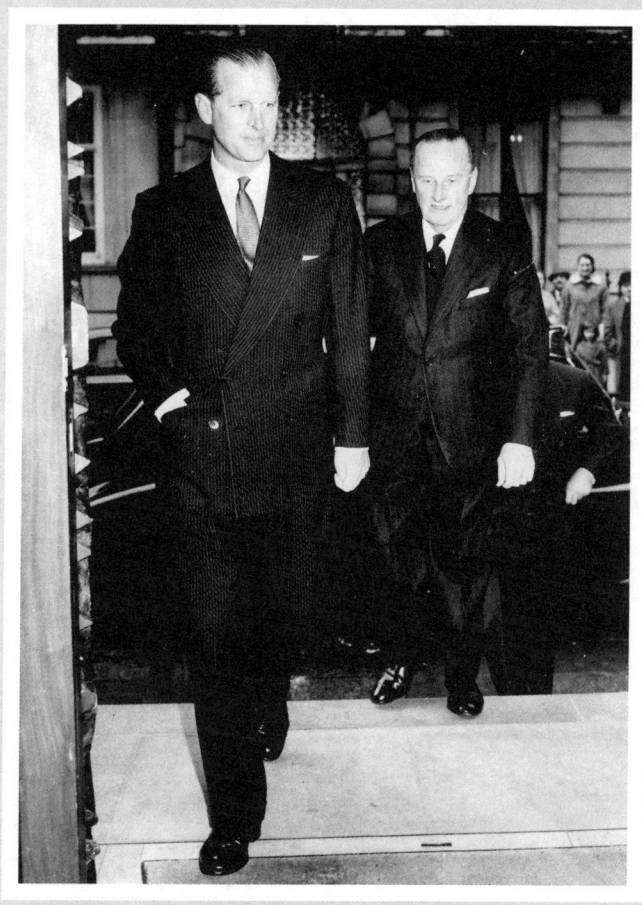

HRH Prince Philip with EWF attending the opening
of the new Council Chamber, General Dental Council

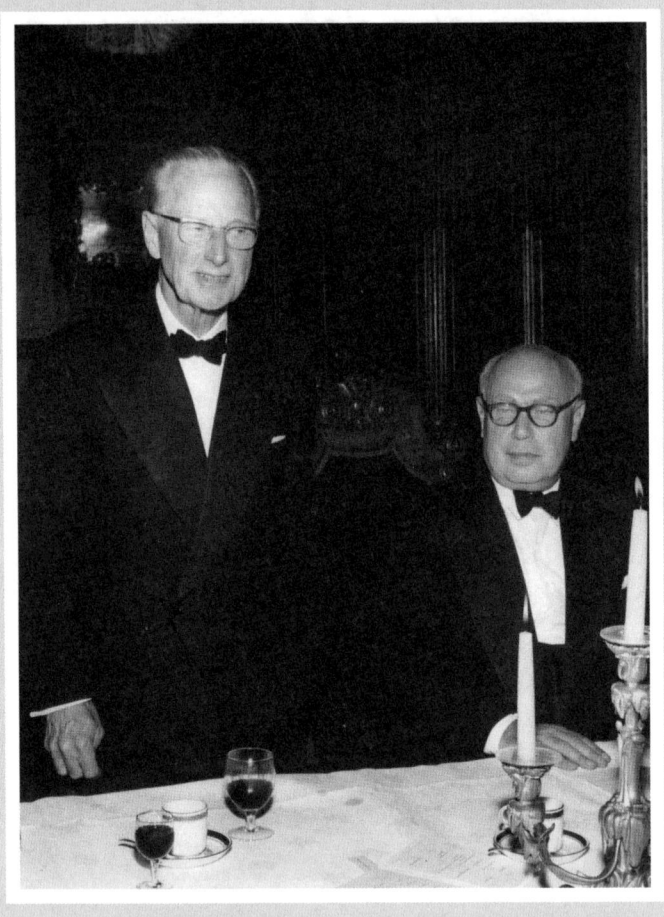

Being dined by the GDC after vacating the
Presidential Chair to Professor Bradlaw on 6th July 1964

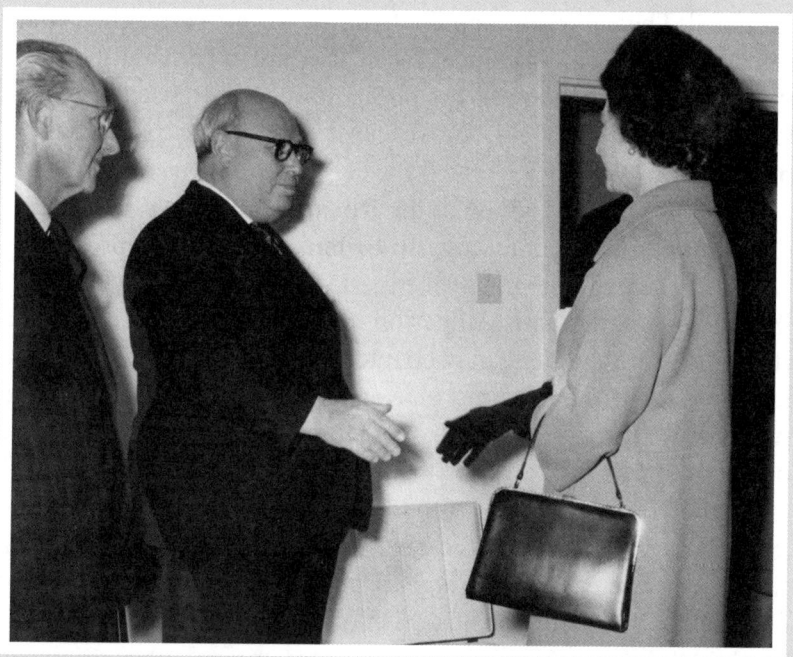

Presentation to HM The Queen at the opening of BDA House, 1968

Chapter 10

PERIODONTAL DISEASE

When in retirement Fish was asked which of all the fields in which he worked gave him the greatest sense of achievement, he answered, "Oh undoubtedly, periodontia .. it was a problem of basic pathology, and in those days ... one had to start from scratch." That was his approach in all his research; he would refer back to basic biological facts. It is not surprising therefore that in the Introduction to his book, 'Parodontal Disease', which was published in 1944, he discusses the basic properties of protoplasm.

In 1932 Fish had set up at the Royal Dental Hospital the first department of periodontology in Britain. The book, representing years of research and practical experience, marked a watershed in the teaching and practise of periodontology, especially in Britain. It begins," Oral hygiene may be interpreted as the care of the gum margins, for if the gum margins are looked after efficiently and maintained in perfect health, the mouth will be clean and the problem of taking care of the teeth will be very much simplified."

In the context of Fish's time, reference to oral hygiene in the introductory sentence to the text marks a radical advance. At a time when the causes of gingival inflammation and periodontal destruction were still debated, Fish was laying down a marker.

Epidemiological studies of disease prevalence produced enormous variation in findings. In England and Wales about forty percent of children were found to have gingivitis, but in Scotland, Sweden, New York and other places the figures were higher, reaching virtually one hundred percent in India. Why such differences? 'Racial' variation was an obvious explanation. Notions of race featured prominently in so many areas of medicine and anthropology in those days.

Some authorities held that boys were more susceptible than girls; others that there was an inverse correlation between dental caries and gingival disease.

The main cause of these apparent variations lay in the lack of well defined criteria for assessing disease. When well defined indices were applied it became generally acknowledged that differences in oral hygiene practice, nutrition, general health, and socio-economic factors were responsible for the differing pictures of disease.

In the early days of the twentieth century the prevalence and severity of periodontal destruction was more difficult to assess because radiographic facilities for the examination of alveolar bone were not available, nor even probes for the careful measurement of the periodontal pocket. Even by the nineteen-fifties reliable epidemiological studies were rare, and one study of gingivitis in children even assumed that some gingival inflammation was normal to children. When Fish turned his attention to periodontal disease, theories of causation abounded. Each small variation in the clinical picture, e.g. colour, swelling, tissue texture, presence or absence of bleeding or pus, provided its particular explanation.

Although the relationship between periodontal disease and the bacterial products of poor oral hygiene did not receive the attention that it did later, one very early observer suspected that there was a connection.

Anthony Von Leeuwenhoek in 1683 wrote in a letter to Francis Aston, Secretary of the Royal Society:

" 'Tis my wont of a morning to rub my teeth with salt, and then swill my mouth out with water; and often, after eating, to clean my back teeth with a toothpick, as well as rubbing them hard with a cloth: wherefore my teeth, back and front, remain as clean and white as falleth to the lot of few men of my years, and my gums (no matter how hard the salt be that I rub them with) never start bleeding. Yet not withstanding my teeth are not so cleaned thereby, but what there sticketh or groweth between some of my front ones and my grinders …. a little white matter….On examining this I judged….. that there yet were living animalicules therein."

In this letter Van Leeuwenhoek seems to suggest a relationship between the absence of animalicules, that is good oral hygiene, and gingival health, but while it might imply a cause and effect relationship it does not prove it. It is also possible to infer from this statement that regular gingival massage, with or without salt, helps to increase keratinisation, toughen the gingivae and thus protect the tissues from the assault of sharp food particles. Fish was familiar with Leeuwenhoek's work, which according to Professor Cohen, he frequently quoted. Fish's description of the pathogenesis of periodontal is therefore not so surprising.

Prior to Fish's research two questions exercised people in the field. First, the cause of gingival inflammation, and then the relationship of that inflammation to destruction of the deeper periodontal tissues, the periodontal ligament and alveolar bone.

The eminent dental teacher, J.F. Colyer, with whom Fish worked after World War I, wrote in 1893 that chronic periodontitis may start near the tooth apex or the free margin (of the gum) in which it is caused by tartar, ligatures (around teeth as in the immobilisation of broken jaws), ... as well as syphilis, anaemia and rheumatism as predisposing causes. Subsequently he wrote that periodontitis was associated with a blow, ligatures around teeth, and collection of food debris in approximal spaces. In these descriptions he seems to be conflating two forms of periodontal inflammation, that is acute inflammation following physical trauma or presenting an acute abscess often the consequence of pulp disease, and chronic periodontitis (pyorrhoea alveolaris or Riggs Disease) in which teeth are gradually loosened and finally lost. Part of the problem was the difficulty in very neglected mouths of distinguishing the specific causal factors which produced the presenting clinical features. Chronic periodontitis, Colyer writes later, " consists in a progressive destruction of the tooth socket sometimes in earlier stages but almost always in later stages by a free discharge of pus from the gum margin........ The disease is widely distributed throughout the human race and in animals under domestication and wild animals kept in captivity..... the gingival margin is a mass of cells, lymphoid in character."

At a meeting of the Royal Society of Medicine in 1913,

Colyer declared that he knew "no means of curing periodontal disease except by free extractions."

One of the earliest microscopic examinations of decalcified sections of periodontal tissues was carried out by Znamensky who found that in all sections a deposit of calculus was present under the gum margin, and " sections showed that the pathological process was of an inflammatory character originating in the gum and leading to the destruction of the periodontal membrane and the adjacent bone."

Calculus, either by physical irritation or by its association with oral debris, was regarded by many as the principal cause of gingival inflammation. G.V.Black, the great American teacher, believed that the presence of calculus prevents the natural stimulus of the gum margin that is caused by the friction of food, therefore its deposition had to be retarded. He recommended restricting the intake of food and treating the bowels with saline laxatives. Even as late as 1948 H.H. Stones, a contemporary of Fish at Manchester, suggested that calculus deposits should be controlled by eating hard food.

At that time Germany led the field in many areas of medicine, and Vienna was a major site of dental research. Bernhard Gottlieb of Vienna is one of the most famous names in this field. He had considerable influence on Fish, who recorded his debt to Gottlieb in the preface to 'Parodontal Disease.'

"I have to acknowledge my debt to Professor Gottlieb for his gift of sections to me many years ago before I had any of my own. I am particularly grateful to him for first arousing my special interest in the pathology of this universal malady."

Gottlieb, who can be regarded as the father of periodontal research, was the first person to describe and appreciate the significance of the 'epithelial cuff' that rings the tooth and seals the tooth root and supporting periodontal tissues from the mouth.. He called it 'Der Epithelanzatz am Zahne' or 'Epithelial Attachment'.

Bernhard Gottlieb was born in 1885 in Poland and in his youth spoke only Hebrew and Yiddish. His potential was recognised early and he was sent to Vienna from where he graduated in 1911 in medicine and dentistry. As a Jew he could not nominally be the Director of the Department of Dental Research, but to all intents and purposes he was just that, and was so regarded by the international community. He demonstrated his practical skills in developing histological embedding in celloidin before paraffin embedding was used. It was from Gottlieb that Fish learnt these new histological techniques.

Professor Alfred Kantorowicz, the author of an encyclopaedia of dentistry and Dean of the dental school in Bonn, tells the story that when Gottlieb applied to take a position at the Bonn school he was told, "One Jew is enough." (Kantorowicz himself being the one).

So Gottlieb stayed in Vienna until 1938 when he and his family fled to Palestine from Nazi persecution. He was invited to a temporary post in Michigan from where he went to Baylor University Dental School as Director of the Dept. of Oral Pathology and Dental Research He died in 1950. Fish had been in correspondence with Gottlieb for many years, and in 1933 he sent him a copy of his book. "An experimental Investigation of Enamel, Dentine and the Dental Pulp". Gottlieb sent a note of thanks, and on that note Fish later wrote," What a tragic life. Damn Hitler."

In Gottlieb's dental anatomy studies he describes the Epithelial Attachment and the normal physiological phenomenon of the "continuous eruption" of the teeth. This told of a synchronisation of changes in the tooth-supporting tissues with age. As teeth wore down with the attrition of use they continued to erupt in order to maintain the vertical dimension of the face, and masticatory function. The gingival margin and epithelial attachment to the tooth moved apically with concomitant atrophy of the alveolar bone margin, while root cementum and apical bone deposited.

Periodontal disease, he believed, represented a distortion of this process in which there was failure of cementum deposition. This resulted in detachment of periodontal fibres from the root surface thus allowing the epithelial attachment to grow down the root to produce the periodontal pocket.

In later writing Colyer says that he always taught that periodontal disease starts as a marginal gingivitis from where it spreads to deeper tissues, a belief supported by the histological work of James and Counsell. But the Canadian, H.K. Box, was convinced that in chronic periodontal disease alveolar rarefaction preceded gingivitis. He believed that the primary lesion was not in the bone or cementum but in the periodontal membrane which provokes secondary resorption of bone via a reaction around the blood vessels. He points to the similarity between 'rarefying pericementitis fibrosa' and osteitis fibrosa, a metabolic disease, and concludes "the lesion of the periodontal membrane is the result of some systemic disturbance rather than a local condition."

The confusion stemmed in part from the idea that the many variations in clinical features represented different forms of the disease, and at that time variation could be striking and difficult to explain. The accumulated burden of poverty, ill-health, malnutrition, compounded by endocrine changes, and very poor oral hygiene together with any intercurrent disease, affected tissue response to infection and irritation. Such response could be acute and florid. It is hardly unexpected that Box classified gingivitis into thirteen varieties.

Fish expressed his frustration with this confusion when he complained about, "the impossibility of applying the exact language of science to such speculative matter is necessarily irritating." Fish like many of his contemporaries was trying to bring dentistry into the modern scientific world, but there were occasions when efforts at precision could be confusing. In the section on periodontal disease in the sixth edition of Colyer and Sprawson's big and popular teaching text there is a footnote:

"The word periodontal literally means, 'around a tooth' but in ordinary technical usage this word is so universally taken to indicate the immediate surroundings of a tooth (the periodontal membrane) that periodontitis has come to mean inflammation of the membrane. The disease which is the subject matter of this chapter does not start or finish as an inflammation of the periodontal membrane, but extends beyond it and involves also bone and gingivae, so that paradontal is a more distinctive and accurate term, covering as it does, all the tissues involved."

In the face of such authoritative pedantry, what could a dental student do but take it on board to be regurgitated at oral examinations.

Fish himself expressed his objection to the prefix peri-; the lesion which he believed started and mainly involved the interdental tissues could not be so described.

Lack of scientific explanation also led to a proliferation of classifications of the disease, all meant to help the student, but which were as meaningful as the Rosetta stone to most readers. Fish agreed with Colyer in his description of the disease as progressive from the initial gingivitis, and he divided the disease into three stages, Phase1 Marginal Gingivitis, Phase 2 Pyorrhoea Simplex, and Phase 3 Pyorrhoea Profunda.

Fish argued that two questions needed to be considered: first, whether the 'parodontal syndrome' could be regarded as a constitutional disease with local symptoms or as one of entirely local origin, and secondly , how does the disease start? In answering the first question he pointed out that the disease responded rapidly and consistently to local treatment, and that people with quite advanced parodontal breakdown could be healthy in every other respect. However, he did note that some people seem to be especially susceptible to the disease, that it can appear early in life, progress rapidly, and recur after treatment. He concluded that "It is quite reasonable to accept as a working hypothesis that the disease is a direct response to local irritation but that there are constitutional factors which make some people more prone to its onset than others and that these same factors , or perhaps others, make them less resistant to its progress and more liable to a recurrence". Over half a century on no-one could dispute that statement.

In ' Parodontal Disease', Fish described the gingival margin in health with emphasis on its "firm keratinous cuticle" and it is this keratinisation which he believed to be crucial to gingival health.

His interest in keratinisation of the gingiva was stimulated at his visit to Australia in 1935 where he received an Honorary DDS from the University of Melbourne. One of his hosts, Harold Vernon Mattingley, had studied the dental condition of the Aborigine population, and his writings attracted Fish's attention. (K.V. Mattingley, writes about his father, H.V. in his book, "Dentist on a Camel", where Fish is mentioned).

On his return to London, Fish wrote to H.V. Mattingley from 31 Queen Anne St., " I hasten to tell you what a profound interest the men in London have shown in your material. I think there is more to be learnt on dental matters from the teeth and bone of the Aborigines than from any other race in the world......You gave me a wonderful time in Melbourne."

Subsequently Fish wrote, "It is delightful of you to let me have all this material. I shall be talking on my Australian experiences in June and shall incorporate your findings. Your record is exactly what I want. I am quite satisfied that there is some factor in the structure of the teeth which renders them relatively immune or less susceptible apart altogether from their environment, but I do not think it is a dietetic factor, that is vitamins and so on , but more the question of hereditary texture, such as the crystallographic arrangement in the enamel."

In this letter Fish was referring to the relative absence of dental caries in Aborigine teeth, but he was equally impressed by their healthy periodontal condition "The reason the savage has hard gums is twofold. For one thing he never has a long "clinical crown" because he grinds away the occlusal surface at about the same rate as the gum margin recedes down the tooth, so that the teeth remain mere studs ground almost level with, and streamlined into, the horny gum margins. Secondly, by "hard" food one does not mean crisp biscuits. The savage does not get starch by swallowing a highly cultivated potato, or even a crisp biscuit, but by chewing for hours on some refractory substance such as the stalk of a young tree fern.....", and as an injunction to the British dentist: the first thing to make clear to the patient is that the soft diet of civilized man does not provide sufficient friction to keep the gum margins hard and firmly keratinized any more than clerical work makes the hands hard like those of a bricklayer. It follows that the gum margins being soft are easily torn by occasional rough sharp particles in the food, and the abrasions so caused often become chronic because of course they are liable to be torn open again at every meal."

"These persistent minute raw places or "ulcers" permit toxic products to diffuse in amongst the fibres which attach the tooth to the jaw - the parodontal fibres.... so that they break away ... working slowly down from those at the gum margin towards those at the apical end of the tooth." He continues, " ... if his food were suddenly made really hard he could not chew it at all, and it would tear his gums if he tried; that is thought to be one reason why the men in the trenches get trench mouth. Some aviators who came down amongst the aborigines of Australia would have starved to death had not the natives obligingly chewed the tough native diet of kangaroo flesh for them."

Here encapsulated is Fish's theory of the aetiology and pathogenesis of the disease. Without keratinisation there is ulceration of the gum margin, and the ulcer allows ingress of bacteria and toxins.

A further aspect of the problem that received Fish's attention was the importance of the interdental morphology:

"In young people the gingival margins are firmly attached to the enamel right up to the contact points of the teeth and there are no interdental spaces. In a very short time, however, detachment inevitably takes place and....... a fine probe may be passed through between each contact point and the gum margin. From this moment onwards this space must receive the attention of both the dental surgeon and the patient." The interdental gingiva, which was to be described in detail by Bertram Cohen, who in 1960 became the first Nuffield Research Professor of Dental Science at the Royal College of Surgeons of England, was labelled by Fish with a mountaineering term, 'the col' because of its shape. Everest had recently been conquered and the col, a depression between the peaks of the lingual and labial papillae, was a familiar shape to everyone. This is not only an area sheltered from stimulus, it is also the site of food and bacterial stagnation. In Cohen's theory of the pathogenesis of periodontal disease the base of the col is particularly vulnerable when there is a breach in the continuity of oral epithelium between one peak of the col and the other; this may arise developmentally if oral epithelium should fail to replace the fragile embyonic reduced enamel epithelium, or subsequently as a consequence of interdental injury.

In short, Fish believed that civilised man should avoid gum disease by toughening the gums, that is increasing keratinisation by regular massage with a toothbrush, and paying special attention to the gum between the teeth with the use of special sticks initially made from balsa wood, the dental wood stick.

Fish's writing on this matter is persuasive, as always in his teaching, it is full of supporting anecdote and analogy, and his suggestion was received with enthusiasm by the profession and by the manufacturers of dental wood sticks. But the technique had its limitation where teeth were tight together and there was little or no dental embrasure. His suggestion of prophylactic 'papillectomy' to produce an embrasure space, was a step too far for most people. Also many people objected to the black interdental triangle that the procedure produced. Occasionally vigorous and careless use of the woodsticks dislodged crowns, which discouraged some folk from continuing their use, and some dentists from recommending the exercise in the first place.

In acknowledging the importance of bacteria and their toxins in producing tissue damage, Fish notes:

"It is not possible to prevent the presence of micro-organisms in the sulcus around the teeth any more than one can prevent lichen on the bark of an old oak tree; the important thing is to prevent both them and their poisons from gaining access to the tissues. It is hopeless to try to clean them away; the only defence is to harden the surface so that they can do no harm."

In his view the presence of the gingival ulcer as the portal of entry for bacteria is essential. His explanation for this is spelt out in his extensive 1935 paper, in which he sets out his understanding of the aetiology and pathogenesis of periodontal disease.

As he does in many discussions about tissue behaviour he goes back to first principles.

Signs of inflammation in the sub-epithelial connective tissue must be caused by one of three types of irritation, mechanical, chemical and physical, and infective.

"It is almost safe to say that the chronic irritant is at first mechanical..., since the epithelium is at first completely intact over these patches of cellular infiltration so that neither chemical nor bacterial irritants could reach the connective tissue concerned."

This statement is vital to an appreciation of his point of view. He could not know that bacterial products can diffuse through epithelium, keratinised or not; indeed the degree of keratinisation seems to be irrelevant to the passage of small molecules. Fish's woodstick regime worked because it cleaned the interdental space and proximal tooth surfaces, not because it induced papillary keratinisation.

About this time the oral flora was being examined in more depth, and animal experiments had shown that infection could result from the normal oral flora. Thus Rosebury wrote that " the severity and duration (of inflammation) depends upon pre-existing tissue changes such as those resulting from local irritation, trauma and occlusal disharmony." Although the flora of soft deposits on the teeth had been shown to be toxic the specific importance of the bacteria was not fully recognised and spelled out. The physical irritation to the gingiva as the edge of calculus deposits rubbed the soft tissue was still regarded as important. One obstacle to the ready acceptance of bacteria as the prime causal agent was the failure of research to fulfil Koch's postulates, i.e. that the specific organism from the lesion could produce another lesion which demonstrated the presence of the same organisms. Other infectious diseases such as diphtheria and tuberculosis fulfilled the criteria, but attempts to induce periodontal disease by the introduction of oral bacteria into the gingivae failed. Further, the idea that disease might be caused by resident bacteria when immunity was impaired, as for example when an intercurrent disease was imposed, was not yet considered. Also the notion that time and bacterial accumulations were essential to the production of inflammation, was not tested, and it was left to other workers, in particular the Scandinavians, Jens Waerhaug and Harald Loe and their colleagues, to demonstrate the role of 'bacterial plaque'.

The need for the surgical elimination of the 'periodontal pocket', the site of bacterial accumulations inaccessible to toothbrush and wood stick, in the treatment of the disease, had been recognised for a long time. With his usual enthusiasm Fish's teaching reinforced the need for gingivectomy, the elimination of the pocket wall "by surgical means, using an appropriately fashioned knife". He had of course designed such knives, which no dental surgeon worth his salt could be without. It seems that MacRoss had some explanation to do when the income tax inspector found the purchase of Fish knives in the practice expense accounts.

Fish's 'Parodontal Disease' is a model of clarity, an expression of the way he brought to bear his understanding of tissue behaviour to its manifestation in the clinical picture. He did all the line drawings himself, which is not surprising from the winner of the Kingswood School prize for Mechanical Drawing. Most of the microscopic slides and microphotographs were prepared by his excellent technician, William Pereira, who himself went on to do medicine; others were given by Bernhard Gottlieb.

There had been many workers in the field before Fish, but his work and teaching were a milestone in our understanding of this almost universal disease, or group of diseases. We now realise that although oral bacterial represent the common aetiological factor, the variation in the clinical and histological features described by Fish represent fundamental variations in the tissue response.

A revised and enlarged edition of 'Parodontal Disease' came out in 1952, in which Fish considers the role of "disharmony of the occlusal relationship". He discounts the idea that occlusion plays a part in the initiation of the disease, for which he finds no evidence, but its role in affecting the progress of disease justifies his detailed discussion of the importance of splinting in periodontal treatment. Another subject receives greater attention in this edition, and that is collagen, and it is not surprising that when a few years later, the biochemist, Dr. John Eastoe, was recruited to Fish's team at the Department of Dental Science at the RCS, it was on the basis of his expertise in this field. Professor Albert Neuberger, the Editor of the Biochemical Journal, was a colleague of Fish's at St.Mary's Hospital, and knowing about Fish's requirements, suggested that Eastoe would fit the bill. His appointment at the Department of Dental Science was to last twenty-three very productive years.

Chapter 11

E.W.F. AND A DEVELOPING PROFESSION

On December 5th. 1910, the year that Fish started his professional training at Manchester Dental School, the case of Mr. and Mrs. Collins versus the Nottingham 'Hygienic Institute', appeared before Belper County Court in Nottingham. The case wonderfully illustrates some aspects of dental practice in Britain. It seems that two men jumped over the Collins' garden wall and introduced themselves as experienced dentists extolling the benefits of treatment by their Institute. They said that they could make Mrs. Collins good false teeth for £3. So persuaded, the lady had four teeth extracted there and then, no doubt without anaesthesia of any sort, and some days later, despite her doctor's advice that only four teeth be extracted at one time, another twelve teeth were removed. After a suitable interval for the gums to heal, dentures were made which were not satisfactory. Nor were a second and third set, because, as she complained, the upper denture dropped when she opened her mouth. In court the judge asked her to open her mouth to witness this unsatisfactory outcome. The Collins won their case, obtaining £3 10s for the false teeth, £3 15s for the doctor's bill, £5 for expenses incurred in buying extra food during Mrs.Collins' illness, and £5 in damages.

At that time the public were exploited by the unqualified, the unregistered, the untrained and by quacks. Such practice was rife, and unfortunately the public did not seem to distinguish the registered from the unregistered dentist. As Muriel Spencer points out in her essay on Robert Lindsay, the first full-time secretary of the BDA, this widespread ignorance or lack of concern promoted extensive malpractice which did nothing to maintain the social status and public esteem of the profession, and in turn led to a shortage of recruits.

Concern was not limited to the BDA and qualified members of the profession. In 1916 the General Medical Council moved that "it is urgently necessary in the public interest that steps be taken to amend the Dentists Act (of 1878) in order that the public may be the better enabled to distinguish qualified from unqualified practitioners of dentistry." Sir Donald MacAlister, President of the GMC, wrote, "The State cannot afford to allow the health of the workers to be continuously undermined by dental neglect."

But there was another and very different aspect to dentistry at that time, and one in which Fish came to play an increasingly influential part. This was one in which professional skills often of a high order, and scientific ideas were applied to clinical practice. This aspect was represented largely by those practitioners with a formal qualification, by national bodies such as the BDA, and collectively by the International Medical Congress and the International Dental Congress, organisations established in the nineteenth century, and of which qualified dentists were a part. At the Eleventh Medical Congress there came the first signs of a schism between the 'odontologists' and the 'stomatologists', the latter insisting on a medical qualification. At that time most of the British delegates to the Congress were doubly qualified.

In 1900 at the 3rd. International Dental Congress, the Federation Dentaire Internationale or FDI was first proposed. This organisation was the brain-child of Charles Godon, Dean of the Ecole Dentaire de Paris, and essentially a breakaway organisation of the Odontological Section of the International Medical Congress. Its function was to represent all dentistry and overlook all aspects of the profession without distinction of nationality. As a reaction to this development the 1913 International Medical Congress held in London banned dentists, who had previously been welcome. The idea that dentists had the temerity to form their own international body could not be stomached by many but not all stomatologists. A few supported the formation of the FDI.

The first London Dental Congress held in August 1914 should have been a joint meeting of the BDA and the Federation, but was frustrated by the imminent outbreak of the war.

The war demonstrated that dental health was a vital part of the general health of an efficient soldier, and that simply providing full dentures to a man rendered edentulous was not the best way forward. Sir Charles Tomes, who was later recruited to the GMC, summed up the situation and at the same time grasped the nettle when he said, "..the present state of things (is) well nigh intolerable... the numbers upon the existing Register are greatly inadequate... the numbers of recognised practitioners shall be largely and immediately increased. This can only be done by according some recognition to those who have been in practice long enough for it to be assumed that they have acquired some measure of knowledge and skill; five years of bone fide practice is suggested as an appropriate time."

The remedy was legislation. The Privy Council set up a committee under the chairmanship of Sir Francis Dyke Acland to amend the 1878 Act, and in 1919 it published a detailed survey of the horrifying state of dentistry in Britain, reporting that "very great evils were associated with the practice of dentistry and dental surgery by persons not qualified under the Dentists Act....in consequence there was a great shortage of registered dentists." It recommended that the law be altered "to prohibit the practice of dentistry by the unregistered "Also it was noted that registered practitioners were very unevenly distributed geographically, and more commonly settled in well populated areas where higher fees were obtainable.

Robert Lindsay was one of those that played a considerable part in the planning, drafting and promotion of the Dentists Act of 1921 under which the practice of dentistry was to be restricted to dentists already registered under the 1878 Act, registered medical practitioners and to a very limited extent, to registered pharmacists. Unregistered dentists of some years standing could also be registered on application. This provision included members of the Incorporated Dental Society (formerly the Incorporated Society of Extractors and Adaptors of Teeth Limited, representing the interests of unqualified men) of over one-year standing, (and some others without qualification). All hopefuls must apply within a given time limit if they were to be eligible for entry to the Register. The Dental Board of the United Kingdom of thirteen members was set up under the chairmanship of Sir Francis Dyke Acland, as a sub- committee of the GMC.

This latter body was confused about its obligations, and initially resented the burden that the government had forced upon it. After all, as comment in the BMJ made clear, "the GMC has not a dentist upon it ... Medicine is a profession ... Dentistry is a business." However its obligations were made clear, they were to approve any recommendation proposed by the three Dental Board members appointed to sit on the Council when dental business was on the agenda. By then Norman Bennett had replaced Charles Tomes on the GMC. He had been appointed by the Representative Board of the BDA to speak on behalf of the BDA and on behalf of the whole profession. Inevitably there were protests about " the evils of unqualified practice" from those with a dental diploma, but the Lancet expressed the general feeling when its editorial endorsed the act in promoting research into the cause of dental caries and providing a service which "should bring within the reach of the working classes treatment such as in many districts has been out of their reach hitherto, except as a matter of charity". The press generally supported the government recommendations, and the Dentists Act 1921 passed through parliament easily.

Applications for registration poured in. The £5 registration fee represented one of the main aggravations, especially as dentists already on the Register did not need to pay. A further complaint was that the lowest age of registration had been set at twenty-three, which excluded younger men who had served as dentists in the armed forces.

The amending Act of 1923 extended the time allowed for registration, and lowered the age of entry to twenty-one. By 1924 there were about 13,000 names on the register of which 5,032 held an LDS, 768 registered under the1878 Act and 7,301 under the 1921 Act.

Setting up the Dental Board was a great step forward, an achievement that bore testimony to the foresight of those men who realised that providing a better dental service and enhancing the prestige of the profession, rested on advances in dental education and dental research. Fish was one of those to benefit from the Board's enlightened support of his research.

But many qualified men would not recognise the 1921 men as their professional equals, and the latter's right to membership of the BDA was hotly debated for the next few years. Membership of their professional organisation represented the formalisation of their status, and it seemed to the qualified practitioners that their status was at stake. Professional and social hierarchies were strongly entrenched and zealously defended, and when in 1923 it was suggested that entry to the register might be facilitated by short courses for the LDS examination, Fish was one of those who protested vigorously against any dilution of training. In a letter to the BDJ in May '23 from Buckhurst Lodge, Fish wrote, "Surely if any educational body is desirous of helping these men to serve the community, the important thing is to educate them, not to provide them with an easy diploma and so confuse them utterly with the properly qualified dental surgeon ... It is useless having an act preventing unauthorized dental practice, if, in the process of time, the standard of the authorizing diploma becomes lowered until it ceases to be any guarantee of efficiency."

In the following month he wrote a much stronger letter, "... concessions both as regards the Preliminary examination, general education and the course in dental mechanics, appear to me to be directly conducive to the lowering of our standards of professional education, a result we should deplore," and he goes on to emphasise the idea that " entrants to our profession have attained a state of intellectual discipline that will enable them to profit by the new matter that is to be laid before them in their professional studies." Fish had in mind a continuing accumulation of knowledge about dental diseases, and the development of new techniques, and writes that, "if a man has attained the age of twenty-five he will have lost much of the receptive power of the child's mind." And he insists that they must have evidence of at least 4 years of approved instruction in dental mechanics, not at the hands of unqualified operators. These letters represented Fish's first appearance on the public stage.

A further subject of concern to the profession, and of particular objection from the BDA, was the employment by school dental clinics of 'dental dressers' who assisted dentists in inspections and charting, and in providing simple dressings, fillings and scalings "under close supervision of the dentist." In defending their employment the Local Education Authority of Sheffield pointed out that its clinics looked after 74,000 children, and its three dressers were essential. It was also pointed out that in the Poor-Law schools where oral hygiene instruction was provided by nurses there had been a big improvement in dental health. Dental wagons with nurses as dressers travelled around rural areas. The Dental Board also expressed anxiety about "the insidious dangers" associated with the employment of dressers. If dentistry was going to become a respected profession it had to be regulated, and seen to be subject to as strict discipline as the GMC imposed on the medical profession. The Dental Board was still a client body of the GMC on whose premises it held its meetings.

Unregulated practice persisted, especially by non-registered assistants to registered men, and in 1924 Sir Leslie Mackenzie, the Crown nominee for Scotland on the GMC, asked Chief Constables for their co-operation in acting against those not on the Register. Advertising and commercialism presented the Dental Board with a considerable problem, and it expressed anxiety about the "list of bodies corporate carrying on 'the business of dentistry'". The editorial of the BDJ expresses disgust at these practices. The Dental Board operated to very strict rules and even struck off the Register practitioners who were late paying the fee, and in reply to those objecting to the high fee of £5 (which was later reduced to £4), pointed out that these fees supported research and provided bursaries and loans to dental students. The Board saw education as one of its primary purposes. Postgraduate courses were provided in amongst other subjects the growth of the jaws, the still mysterious matter of periodontal diseases, and the critically important subject, dental anaesthesia. Death following general anaesthesia was all too common. The Board demonstrated its forward-looking thinking by producing films for young people on oral hygiene and care of the teeth.

In the research for his MD, a report of which had appeared in the BDJ in 1924, Fish had made clear the hazards of local anaesthetics, and almost immediately on the completion of his thesis he had started his research on the lymph supply of the dentine and enamel, for which he was a recipient of a research grant from the Board. His report on this work first appeared in the BDJ in 1927. That was the year in which Mr. Eastman proposed to provide a Dental Dispensary for the District of London. Eastman recognised that prevention of disease is much more important than treatment, and had in 1915 already established in the USA the first Eastman Dental Clinic with provision for maternity and child welfare, and for the treatment of tonsils, adenoids and cleft palates.

The Eastman Clinic was to be added to the Royal Free Hospital, "a well-known training ground for medical women." But it was made clear from the outset that this extension of the Royal Free was not going to be a school for training women dentists.

This was also the year in which Fish became a new and enthusiastic member of the British division of the Scientific Research Commission of the F.D.I. He brought forward a resolution proposed earlier by Dr. Bernhard Gottlieb, then the Chairman of the Research Commission, that a competition be held to test experimentally the effectiveness of root canal treatment. In his enthusiasm, Gottlieb had already opened a subscription to support the competition before the FDI executive had authorised him to do so. In the event the public announcement of a competition in which animal experimentation would be involved raised such a storm in the press and from animal rights movements that no one entered for the competition. It was left to Fish in the Hampton Hale Laboratory to carry out Gottlieb's suggested experiment.

In accordance with the Dental Board's requirements for the continuation of his research grant Fish made regular progress reports which were to satisfy the MRC's Committee for the investigation of dental disease. In 1928 Fish had visited Gottlieb in Vienna, there to learn the technique of preparing celloidin sections for his research on dentine and enamel. This was to start a relationship of mutual respect that Fish valued and always acknowledged.

St. Mary's Hospital

In May 1928 W.H.Dolamore FRCS, LRCP, LDS resigned from his position as Honorary Dental Surgeon to St. Mary's and was made Consulting Dental Surgeon to the hospital. This was an honour roughly equivalent to that of Emeritus Professor and one which was well deserved. In a long and distinguished career Dolamore had been Dental Surgeon to the Westminster and London Hospitals as well as to St. Mary's. He had been the Dean of the Royal Dental Hospital School of Dental Surgery, President of the BDA, and one-time editor of the British Journal of Dental Science. He was also appointed in 1921 one of the first members of the Dental Board and served as Chairman of the GMC Dental Education and Examinations Committee. Like all the 'Honoraries' of his time, and many 'Hospital Consultants' after the institution of the NHS in 1948, he ran a thriving practice.

The posts Dental Surgeon and Assistant Dental Surgeon were not onerous, their hospital commitment often being only half a day a week largely unpaid. The dental clinics were run by full-time salaried Clinical Assistants with an LDS qualification, frequently women. Most hospitals were independent charities, Voluntary Hospitals supported by legacies, bequests, endowments and subscriptions as well as by donations from the Hospital Governors. Benefactors to St. Mary's included assurance companies, Boots the Chemists, Selfridges, the railway companies, and in 1930 Two Thousand Guineas was received from the House of Rothschild. Fish was to receive the support of another Anglo-Jewish benefactor.

Dolamore's position was taken by Herbert Smale, also one-time Dean at the RDH, and Fish was appointed Assistant Dental Surgeon and subsequently in 1940 Dental Surgeon, a post he held until he retired in September 1959. Thus he served the hospital in a clinical capacity for a period of over thirty years, but apart from improving the facilities of the dental surgery his clinical activity goes largely unrecorded. On the other hand his research work at the Meyerstein Dental Research Laboratory which he founded, was important. This laboratory was set up in an unoccupied part of the third floor of St. Mary's Hospital next to the Inoculation Department, the director of which was Alexander Fleming's predecessor, the famous bacteriologist, Sir Almroth E.Wright, the subject of one of Fish's many eponymous lectures. Almroth Wright was one of the first people to consider specific immunity and his work on wounds during the 1914-18 war had convinced him that many of the antiseptics and disinfectants then in use did more harm to the body defences than the bacteria. Fleming had been his co-worker, and with Wright believed that bacteria had to be fought with weapons specifically lethal to them alone. This principle underlay Fleming's pursuit of his observation in 1928 that the action of a stray mould, Penicillium-P Notatum, inhibited growth of a plate culture of staphylococci in his laboratory. Fish working in the neighbouring laboratory, was one of those first to see this phenomenon.

Some of the work that Fish considered his most important, that on oral streptococci, was carried out with the collaboration of the bacteriologist, Dr. I.H. MacLean.

Subsequently Fleming and Fish collaborated on the use of penicillin in oral and dental infections. They were to become friends, going dancing together with their wives. They also played billiards together at the Chelsea Arts Club where Fleming was also an honorary member.

Fish's benefactor, Edward William Meyerstein (1863-1942), was a highly successful member of the London Stock Exchange and a great philanthropist. Indeed he was renowned as " the great benefactor of hospitals". He gave the Middlesex Hospital in London a gift of £350,000, which made possible its expansion. Beneficiaries of his generosity included the Queen Victoria College Hospital in Tonbridge, the Kent County Ophthalmic Hospital at Maidstone, and in London the Westminster, St. Mary's and Princess Elizabeth of York hospitals. He served as the High Sheriff of Kent and was knighted in 1938 for his benefactions to health services. Whether he was a patient of

Fish's is not known, but it would not be surprising. Fish was on very good terms with many of his important patients, and never seemed shy of taking advantage of opportunity. Also his enthusiasm for his research work might easily have been passed on to such a willing benefactor as Edward Meyerstein at a time when dental caries and periodontal disease were widespread, their causes still something of a mystery, and Fish prominent in their research.

Apart from his work at the Meyerstein, Fish was carrying out research in two other places, at UCL and at the RDH, and it is sometimes difficult to define which experiment took place where, but the Dental Board report of 1928 lists the following work to which their grants applied.

1) the effect of limiting Vitamin B on the teeth of guinea pigs. This work was in collaboration with Dr. Leslie Harris of the National Nutritional Laboratory in Cambridge.

2) an examination of foetal jaws

3) hypoplastic bands in enamel (with Dr.H.A.Harris at the department of Anatomy, UCL)

4) repeating and extending Gottlieb's work on implanting human root apices into animal muscle, using teeth with vital pulps, gangrenous pulps, and teeth with various root filling materials.

Fish was forging ahead with his work on dentine and enamel, and exchanged a lengthy correspondence in the BDJ with Evelyn Sprawson who was doing similar work at the London Hospital. His lecture load was increasing, his topics as diverse as his research on dentine and enamel, full denture design, and dental anaesthesia. He gave detailed accounts of his research at postgraduate lectures at the RDH. At the same time he was promoting Gottlieb's suggestion for the FDI competition on root-canal therapy. At the 1930 Annual Meeting of the BDA he gave a demonstration with the anaesthetist Dr. Clausen, of oral surgery under general anaesthesia.

By this time the Dental Board was considering "the requirements of dentistry as a department of university education", and discussing whether effective teaching could be carried out "upon the altruistic sacrifices of busy practitioners". The Board came to the conclusion that while part-time teachers could still be useful in some subjects whole-time teachers were chiefly needed for "dental surgery, orthodontics, and allied clinical subjects". This was sufficiently vague to leave honoraries undisturbed, but the days of specialisation in clinical subjects were on the horizon. Specialisation had already taken place in pre-clinical subjects such as anatomy, physiology and bacteriology, with striking advances in those areas. The Board concluded that there was "demand for specialisation in the art of imparting and inculcating the application of science no less than in teaching its theory." The practical application of these words had yet to be worked out, but the writing was on the wall and all-rounders like Fish were very slowly to be replaced, but that would take another quarter of a century and another war to eventuate.

In those years Fish continued to be busy, and his activities were not restricted to Britain. In 1931 Fish was a founding member of the London Division of the International Association of Dental Research (IADR), and became President of the Research Commission of the FDI, a position he held for five years, and which brought him into greater contact with European colleagues.

During these years the shadow of the Nazis fell increasingly on the many dental teachers and research workers who were Jewish, and the flight from Germany and Austria started. Professor Alfred Kantorowicz, then Dean at Bonn, escaped to Switzerland, after having been released from a concentration camp at the intercession of Crown Prince Gustav of Sweden, head of the Red Cross. Then with many other Jewish professors, Kantorowicz was invited by Kemal Attaturk to teach at the University of Istanbul, and at the International Dental Congress of 1936 in Vienna, Kantorowicz was a Turkish delegate. Others had later to flee when the Turks decided that Hitler was going to win the Second World War, but for most refugees Turkey proved a safe haven.

Some of the consequences of the 1921 Dentists Act were

unravelling, including the provision that dentistry could be practised by medical practitioners and chemists. In 1931 the Chemists' Dental Society asked the Dental Board whether there might be special provision for chemists to obtain dental qualifications so that they could practise. It seems not to have been obvious to the formulators of the Act that dentists needed to be specially trained. The Board had no answer for the chemists, nor did it seem had the GMC. The control of dentistry by the medical profession was very vigorously attacked by the President of the Southern Counties Branch of the BDA, V.C. Visick, when he declared, "It was an evil moment when in 1878 dentistry in England was placed under the control of the General Medical Council." He railed against dentistry's unequal terms with the medical profession and "the consequent low esteem in which our profession is held," and compared the English situation with that in America which holds "a premier place in dentistry" and is independent of the medical profession.

Fish had been taking an increasingly active role at the BDA Southern Counties Branch, and became President in 1932. This was to be a decade in which new dental schools were founded in Glasgow, Dundee, Leeds and Newcastle, therefore the status of dentistry and the form of dental education were two of Fish's preoccupations. He was familiar with Visick's views as well as American practice and professional status because he and Visick had just visited Canada together, with Fish lecturing on his work. But in his own Presidential address given in Canterbury, Fish gave his attention to elevating the education of the dental student and thereby the image of the profession. It was a long and eloquent address central to which he asked the questions, "Do we wish to produce mere technicians or cultured men and women. Is our calling to become a matter of manipulative skill or a learned profession? Must we prepare for it at technical schools or at a university?" There is no doubt that Fish regarded much American training, even though it could produce wonderful dentistry, as belonging to the former category. Not long after "an event of some significance in the history of dental education", as the BDJ reported it, occurred. An appointment was advertised for a

Readership in Conservative Dentistry in the University of London tenable at Guy's Hospital Medical School. The response from the dental profession was swift and predictable. The BDJ editorial commented, " the dental school is presumably only an appendage to the medical school ....(there is) something incongruous in attaching ....a teaching post in conservative dentistry to a medical school." Over those years there were constant references in lectures and in the dental press to 'The recognition of dentistry as a profession' and 'The separation of dentistry from medicine', and in 1934 it was pointed out that although there were three representatives of the GMC on the Dental Board there was not a single dentist on the GMC.

In 1933, the year that Hitler became Chancellor of Germany, the BDA Council made a public declaration that it considered it wrong for reasons of race, religion or politics to deprive dentists anywhere of the rights which had been granted to them by diplomas and degrees, and discussed how to help these colleagues. The political climate did not stop the Ninth International Dental Congress of 1936 from going ahead in Vienna. In fact it was attended by about three thousand members and was the first dental congress to have simultaneous translation.

There is no record as to whether Gottlieb made any overtures about finding refuge in Britain, as so many other refugees did. Fish would certainly have supported such an application, but it is very likely that Gottlieb, at the top of the dental research tree, would have balked at fulfilling the requirements then set for registration by the Dental Board. Would a British dental school have found him a place? Interestingly, Professor Kantorowicz, fearing rejection by Turkey, registered himself with the Dental Board, but fortunately never needed British refuge.

The registration of foreign dentists fleeing from Nazi persecution presented the Board with a problem which became more acute towards the end of the 'thirties. Applications for registration came from Germany, Austria, Czechoslovakia and even from a few Italian medical graduates who practised dentistry. In 1938 the German Civil Rights Law of the 25th. July, revoked licence to practise medicine by persons of Jewish blood in Germany and Austria, and the Board received unofficial word that this law also applied to Jewish dentists. Further, no Jew had the right to the titles 'Doctor' and 'Dental Surgeon'. For a time in Vienna Jewish dentists could treat Jewish patients. The situation in Czechoslovakia was uncertain. The Dental Board required documents, that is original diplomas and certificates, which would furnish evidence of entitlement to practise dentistry prior to disentitlement under the law of 25th. July, plus the precise date of disentitlement. Things were not made easy for the refugees. Even if qualifications were recognised it was made clear that this did not imply permission to reside or practise in the UK. The Board was very slow in recommending to the Privy Council the right to registration; thus Wilhelm (Willy) Grossmann, a Prague graduate in medicine and dentistry and already serving as a captain in the RAMC, had to write to the Board as late as 1943 to ask, "When a decision in this matter might be expected?" Gradually many refugees were registered, but most had to re-take examinations regardless of their experience and previous qualifications. Only sixteen German dentists, all medically qualified, were admitted without this requirement. Being doubly qualified Grossman was at last allowed to practise and subsequently became head of the orthodontic department at University College Hospital Dental School. Indeed after the war many refugees built thriving practices in the medical areas of London and other cities. They brought the European ethos of trying to save teeth at all costs, a doctrine to which, with some qualification Fish could subscribe.

Scarcely a year passed without Fish having one or two articles published, either on his work on vitamins, or on prosthetics or oral surgery, and in 1933 he was awarded the J. Howard Mummery prize. Some of his research was carried out at St. Mary's Hospital and some at UCL, and the Hampton Hale laboratory continued to be busy. Indeed it seems to have been the only formal dental research laboratory in Britain.

In 1936 B.G.Bibby, a New Zealander teaching at the Rochester Dental School, of which he later became the Director, visited a number of dental schools in Britain and wrote about his impressions. He was especially critical of teaching and research. "Only a small proportion of teachers hold full-time appointments...students receive the greater part of their instruction at the hands either of dentists who spend the bulk of their time in private practice or of men who have no dental qualification or experience....Research activity in dental schools has not yet assumed any importance...active research is being carried out in one school only." That school was the RDH. Bibby went on to comment that the reason for the paucity of research was "traceable to the absence of any academic body in dentistry, capable of undertaking protracted investigation and to the fact that there is no mechanism for interesting and training dentists for research work."

The need for research and greater activity in public health was obvious, and in an article on 'Dentistry and Public Health' Fish cited the fact that while two and a half million of children's teeth were extracted only one million were filled. Further, the Prudential Approved Society's report stated, "neglect of tooth trouble is the cause of quite half of the ill-health found among the industrial classes." At the Empire Dental Meeting of July 1936, Sir George Newman, the Chief Medical Officer at the Board of Education and Ministry of Health, had stated, "the time seems to have fully come for (Insurance Act) extension. The dental profession cannot, it is true, save the people from dental caries and all its results, but it can, if it will, teach and help the people to save themselves."

Fish was to conclude , "If our nation were free from mouth poisoning it would be the happiest and healthiest on earth."

In the past he had published in the BDJ short reports of his research under the heading Laboratory Research Notes, but in 1938, as well as a letter on the bacteriology of the pulp, Fish published eleven of these Research Notes at almost monthly intervals. The topics covered examples of oral pathology as well as work on tooth tissue and bone. All carried excellent pictures of the histo-pathology of the lesions. In 1939 eleven more Research Notes appeared. No other research worker received a fraction of the coverage for their work, and by then Fish's name must have become a dental household word. It is hardly surprising that in that year he was elected to the Dental Board. What is surprising is the size of his vote. Four candidates had been put up for two places on the Board. The electoral system used was that of the transferable vote; the votes were as follows: E.W.Fish 3,002: W.H.Gilmour 655; C.F.Rilot 481; J.A.Woods 264. Fish and Gilmour were elected to the Board. Fish had received almost three-quarters of votes cast; it is doubtful whether any candidate had before or since received such a resounding vote of confidence from his profession.

A few months later, on Sunday September 3rd., war with Germany was declared. Almost immediately a Dental War Committee formed to "make it possible for the services of the profession to be used to the greatest national advantage."

One of those recruited to advise the government in drawing up plans for treating war injuries was William Kelsey Fry, an Honorary Dental Surgeon to Guy's Hospital and Director of the maxillo-facial injuries unit at East Grinstead Hospital. In the First War he had had a distinguished career, winning the Military Cross, and working with the pioneer plastic surgeon, Harold Gillies, and with Warwick James.

Kelsey Fry became an advisor to the Health Department. He also became a director of the Post-graduate Medical Federation supervising the training of Registrars to become hospital consultants in dentistry; in the following years the path of his career and that of Fish were to coincide in many ways.

Chapter 12

AT THE DENTAL BOARD

At the outbreak of World War II the Dental Board was faced with a situation it had no precedents to refer to; there had been no such board in 1914. It had to maintain the Dental Register and discipline within the profession, as well as act against illegal practise. But its responsibilities to education and research were hampered by lack of funds and manpower. Bursaries to students and the Board's annual grant of £3,000 to the MRC were discontinued. Although dentistry became a reserved occupation and dental students, like medical students, were also reserved, dentists had to register under the National Services (Armed Forces) Act, that is to be available for service. Many dentists had joined up as soon as war was declared, and Major G.S.Jones became in 1940 the first dentist to be awarded the Distinguished Service Order (DSO) for courage at Dunkirk on the night of June 1-2.

Although the crisis of war dominated everyone's mind there was also considerable debate about the future. A motion in the House of Commons proposed a widening of health care by an extension of National Health Insurance to include provision of medical treatment to the dependants of insured people, extending hospital treatment to the whole of the insured population and raising the annual income limits for manual workers from £250 to £420. These provisions would bring 40 million people into the scheme.

In 1941 three members of the Dental Board, A.Cubie, W.H.Gilmour and E.W.Fish wrote a joint communication in the BDJ on dental education. It was a signpost to the future. They pointed out the inadequacies of present training in which dental students were clinical dogs-bodies used by the hospital administration in a desperate attempt to cope with the massive demand for treatment from a population with a very high level of disease and unable to pay for private treatment. The emphasis in the students' day was on extraction and the provision of dentures.

The writers called for the introduction of house-surgeons to deal with the clinical demand so that students had more time to spend on professional training with an extension of academic instruction. More attention had to be paid to "the prevention of disease and the preservation of the dentition."

But the call for change went much further. At that time the form of dental education was controlled by the GMC, and the communication questioned whether " supervision and control of the students' needs could not be better discharged by the Dental Board ....with, of course, still the co-operation of academic representations from the Council." The message was clear. Too much of the attitude of the GMC to dentistry and therefore to dental education was dominated by senior hospital medical clinicians, the Honoraries, who put little value on dental health. The Dental Board had to take responsibility for an extension of the academic instruction of dental students, and grants from the Board "should prove a valuable instrument by providing the dental schools with lectureships and professorial posts of their own in the more general scientific subjects ... without divorcing it from the medical school or from hospital practice." By this time the appointment of full-time teachers and the reorganisation of teaching programmes had resulted in obvious benefits, and there was pressure for part-time teachers to attend more frequently and be reduced in number.

In a subsequent communication Fish wrote, "If the student is taught every branch of dental surgery he will not have time for the continual round of extractions, dentures and plastic fillings...hospitals will have to employ house surgeons and provide house appointments for the newly qualified."

Fish was making his mark in the Board, and in Cubie and Gilmour he had effective allies. Gilmour, as the holder of the first Chair in Dental Surgery in Britain, appointed at Liverpool in 1920, and one of the original Board members of 1921, was highly respected, and Adam Cubie had been a revolutionary tutor at Glasgow Dental School. As a tutor Cubie was the first teacher in Britain to introduce G.V. Black's techniques of cavity preparation, and perhaps even more radically had refused to take on his course in operative dentistry any student who could not produce evidence of having passed the first professional examination in chemistry, physics, anatomy and physiology. Apparently the number of students enrolled at the school fell from 100 to 2, but Cubie had the backing of his Dean and the rest of the staff, and thereby had dealt a severe blow against the spread of unqualified practitioners.

One idea linked all Fish's research and that was that clinical practice must be underpinned and validated by research findings, so it is not surprising that the Board formed a Clinical Investigation Committee with Fish as its Honorary Secretary, to enquire into those lines of research which would be relevant to clinical practice, and to associate this activity with post-graduate education. The other two members of this committee were Cubie and F.J. (Fred) Ballard. Ballard, who had been elected a Board member in 1936, had been one of those who had supported Fish's applications for research funds at a time when Lady Mellanby and her supporters were attacking Fish's research on enamel and dentine. His son, Clifford, was to become Professor of Orthodontics at the Eastman Clinic.

By 1942, the war demanding more manpower resources, the Ministry of Labour and National Service announced an extension of the recruitment of doctors and dentists to the 41-46 age group. Female dental mechanics and dental nurse-receptionists aged 20-30 also became liable for 'transfer'. As more dentists entered the forces the Board's income dropped, and when in that year, W.H.Gilmour died, the Board felt that it could not afford to run an election for his successor. Instead it considered the idea of cooption if that were possible under the regulations, and indeed Professor R. V. Bradlaw was coopted.

Despite wartime restrictions, and perhaps because the difficulties of the war focussed official minds on essentials, the idea of universal health care and with it dental care, came to receive more and accelerating attention. Sir George Newman, the Chief Medical Officer recalled the loss of manpower in the war of 1914-18 due to dental disease, and the Insurance Committee under the national Health Insurance Act reported that "anaemia, gastric troubles, debility, neurasthenia and rheumatism were attributable or aggravated by defective teeth." There was call for the "provision of dental treatment for the industrial classes" and a government spokesman stated, " it becomes clearly manifest that private patients…keep their teeth…while panel patients lose them; the Ministries will not rest until they have secured these same benefits for that section of the community for which they are responsible."

In an article on education in the BDJ, Fish pursued his ideas about the need for research-based academic teaching as essential for good clinical practice, and laid down a blueprint for future dental education. He suggested the establishment of a professorial post in dental pathology, and further suggested that schools must have adequate libraries and museums, and that "professors in clinical subjects should have special qualifications too."

In the same issue of the journal Professor R.V. Bradlaw, who held the Chair of Oral pathology at King's College, Durham University and was Sub-Dean and Director of Dental Studies, considered the dual need for trained dental teachers to fulfil their academic duties in the dental school, and also to provide in the related dental hospital treatment for "that large section of the poor deprived of treatment since there was nowhere else for them to go."

The Ministry of Health appointed an Interdepartmental Committee on Dentistry to which Bradlaw was appointed; this stated that provision was to be made for the inclusion of dental treatment as part of a comprehensive health service. Professor E. Sheridan, the Dental Board's Chairman, in his 1943 address, cited his predecessor, Sir Francis Dyke Acland's description of the Board's situation in 1938 as a "half-way house" to independence from the GMC, when he said, " The house is halfway between the government of the dental profession by the medical profession which has prevailed from 1848 to 1921, and the government of the dental profession by itself."

By then Fish was on three of the six committees of the Board, those of Finance, Education and Research, and Dental Health Education, but still making time to publish and lecture on his current favourite topic, the cause and prevention of periodontal disease. In 1944 he was appointed by the Privy Council to be the Chairman of the Board, as he said later, to supervise the transition to a General Dental Council, which he anticipated would be made without much delay. He was to be disappointed; it would take twelve years.

In his address to the 47th. session of the Board, following his tribute to Sheridan, Fish said, "It has fallen to my lot to be appointed to fill his place, and I have accepted the responsibility with no misapprehension of the magnitude and difficulty of the problems that already beset our path." He announced that the Board had given an account of its activities, and made recommendations to the Interdepartmental Committee chaired by Lord Teviot, in which it proposed a Dental Council separate from that of the GMC, a development that had been predicted by Dyke Acland years earlier. Fish said, "the time has come to take a further step in this direction", but he added a rider, " there should be no misunderstanding about this recommendation, and no mischievous suggestion of a divorce from Medicine."

At about that time Fish received a request from Bryan Wood, then Editor of the BDJ, to submit a paper on his thoughts about the future development of a dental service. Fish set about this task in a preparatory manuscript with the rather ominous title, 'Coming events cast their shadows...' He suggested that as adults, both dentists and in the population at large, were set in their ways, the major priority of the future lay in treating children in school clinics, and training dental students to learn preventive dentistry. In addressing the shortage of dentists he proposed the training of ancillary workers, 'a subordinate grade of operators', who like the New Zealand Dental Nurses, could fill teeth. Also he cited the use of ancillary workers in the RAF, who although not properly registered, already carried out scalings and provided oral hygiene instruction. He went further and proposed that the facilities of school clinics should be extended to young adults, and to expectant and nursing mothers. His most contentious idea was the training of dental technicians as prosthetists.

The whole emphasis of the paper lay in care for the community and adaptation of the dental service to that end. The paper was rejected. Later Fish made a note on the manuscript, "apparently they didn't like it!"

In his Presidential Address to the Board in 1945, just after victory in Europe had been celebrated, Fish continued with his call for independence and proposed to the Interdepartmental Committee on Dentistry that, "each dental school (be) a completely adequate scientific and technical department closely integrated with other scientific and technical departments and faculties of the university." He suggested that teachers of physiology, biochemistry and pathology should have dental knowledge, and devote their whole time to dental students, and he picked up on the theme raised earlier by Bradlaw, that is the collateral obligation of the staff of the dental hospital and students to "maintain a charitable service for the necessitous poor." By coincidence, Bradlaw had just been appointed to the Board to fill a vacancy.

Looking to the implementation of the governments intention to include dental care in a universal health service, Fish pointed to the need for training more teachers to cope with the influx to the profession from the armed services now that the war was over, and he called for the formal training of dental ancillaries in approved institutions. In this he demonstrated a wider view of dental care provision than many in the profession were prepared to accept, expressed especially by some vocal members of the BDA. 'Dilution', that cry of alarm from all professions when ancillary workers enter the ring, had not yet appeared in the vocabulary of the dental profession, but the fear was there. In referring to the financing of the expanding schools, Fish made it clear that although the Board would continue to make grants towards the employment of some staff, the duty of subsidising dental education was not one of the Board's functions.

However since its inception in 1921 the Board had the requirement to spend its surplus funds on public purposes in relation to dental education and research. Fortunately the Board had about £20,000 in a 'general unappropriated reserve', and this went immediately to the schools. Despite the Labour Government's promise of funding, this came through very slowly, and without the support from the Board the number of full-time teachers employed would have been very small. As Fish commented, "bis dat qui cito dat - he gives twice who gives quickly." This burden on the Board's finances did not persist for long because the University Grants Commission took over the responsibility for financing the schools. By the end of the war the sixteen dental schools had three hundred full-time teachers.

It looked as though the aftermath of the war pointed to great changes, and as testimony to the general feeling for social change, a Labour government had been elected in a landslide victory with Clement Attlee as Prime Minister. Michael Foot wrote, "it was a vote for a new world." Aneurin Bevan was appointed Minister of Health.

Churchill still continued to come for treatment, now at 34 Weymouth Street, a large double-fronted house built in the style of the English Domestic Revival popular at the end of the nineteenth century, where Fish, having obtained a lease in January of 1945, then lived and practised. No doubt Fish commiserated with the great man on his defeat by an ungrateful nation. Fish had his own problems at that time, having separated from his wife. But his adult children were no longer dependant, James was in South Africa, and Fish's workload was eased by a home in central London, close to the offices of the Board and not too far from St. Mary's Hospital.

In 1946 there was another sign of that 'new world'; Lilian Lindsay became the first woman President of the BDA. The Minister of Health announced that the Dental Research Committee of the Medical Research Council was to be reconstituted. Interestingly, Bradlaw did not offer himself for election to the Board. It is likely that his work load in Newcastle and on various government committees was already heavy enough, even for someone of his enthusiasm and energy. In his Chairman's address, Fish said," It was not granted to us to enjoy for so long the advantage of Professor Bradlaw's help; but everyone who sat on the Board will hope that the governing body of the dental profession have not heard the last of one of the best intellects and keenest wits that ever adorned our debates."

Robert Vivian Bradlaw was born in Dublin in 1903, graduated in dentistry and medicine at Guy's, and then worked part-time at the RDH where he assisted Fish at the Hampton Hale Laboratory. In 1936 he went to Newcastle as the first holder of the Board funded Chair in Dental Surgery, where his drive expanded the school and put Newcastle on the dental map. At the outbreak of war he was appointed Chairman of the No.1 District Dental War Committee, and from 1939-46 he directed the Maxillo-Facial Centre at Shotley Bridge Hospital. He was one of the most consummate politicians that dentistry has produced, and his presence on any health committee would ensure that the voice of dentistry was heard. He was to work closely with Fish, and as Lady Fish was to comment, they were both men who were determined to get their own way.

In October of 1946, doubtless at Bradlaw's invitation, Fish gave the first Founders and Benefactors Lecture at the Sutherland (Newcastle) Dental School, his theme, The Future of Dentistry. This was a wide-ranging talk that Fish concluded by looking to the teachers of the profession to devise a satisfactory curriculum, and select and train good students. In addressing teachers he said, "We outside your schools can only contrive that you have the tools you need, and the opportunity you desire." Until that time the curriculum and supervision of examinations had been in the hands of the GMC, but in the following year the Council and the Board recommended to the Teviot Committee that these responsibilities should fall to the Board. Fish's work for his profession was recognised in the following year by his being awarded CBE.

On November 6th. 1946 the National Health Service Bill received the Royal Assent.

Its proposal had met with fierce opposition from the medical and dental professions, the only exception being the Socialist Medical Association. The BDA had been in favour of a grant-in-aid system of payment which would allow dentists to set their own fees, and pointed out that the fixed fee system applied to practices with much variation in treatment standards and overheads must encourage speed in working and economy of expenses "neither of which is necessarily concomitant with better dentistry." The regulations for dentists included a list of treatments that could not be carried out without prior approval from the Dental Estimate Board and the BDJ editorial protested that Bevan was "claiming a power over the dentist which he would not dream of claiming over the doctors." However the fees offered were so attractive that as one dentist put it, "I can continue to run my Rolls Royce."

In February 1949 Bevan in the House of Commons was able to say, "Who would have said by now even in the most obdurate of all the professions, the dental profession, we should have got 92% of dentists in it." He went on to say that one and three-quarter million people have applied for free dental treatment since setting up the NHS.

In his Chairman's Address Fish referred to the repercussions of the NHS and the anxiety of the Board in relation to abuse of the scheme. Because of the huge demand for free dental treatment dentists were working long hours and the Board was concerned about the standard of individual professional conduct. He said that, "if a practitioner should accept more patients than can be given his undivided and sustained attention, there will be some work done of a standard which cannot be approved." Also he protested about some patient being accepted for part of the treatment under the scheme and advised to contract privately for the rest. He stated, "it has been an unwritten law in our profession that a dentist should perform each operation to the best of his ability." He went on to condemn dental companies which by their "very nature cannot be other than commercial." His conclusion reflected his anger at these many abuses, "we should no longer be talking of a profession, and the brotherhood of professional men would be no more."

In 1949 the government made a 20% cut in dental remuneration, followed by a 10% cut the next year. The demand for treatment out-stripped all predictions and demonstrated the massive neglect of dental health of previous years.

By 1950 other matters occupied Fish's attention. The GMC had recommended that there should be a period of internship prior to full registration of medical graduates, and Fish recommended a year of hospital work for dental graduates to increase their experience and skill.

Many cases of abuse of the NHS Acts had been brought before the Board and Fish insisted that the Board must exclude from their consideration of cases the result of proceedings of any NHS tribunal or Dental Service Committee. The Board had its own criteria of professional conduct and its own disciplinary procedures.

Fish pointed out that the annual retention fee, which had been reduced during the war, was still £2 2s, but the financial responsibilities of the Board had been reduced because the University Grants Committee now funded the dental schools and the revived Dental Committee of the MRC supported research.

But so far as Fish was concerned the most important event of 1950 was his marriage to Hazel, whose first husband, Francis Hodge, had painted Fish's portrait in his doctorate gown. The portrait was painted in payment of dental treatment. Fish had known the Hodges for many years, and as an unattached man had joined them on painting trips when Hodge taught Fish to paint. After Francis Hodge died, although not yet divorced from his first wife, Fish's friendship with Hazel blossomed. Even though they had known each other for many years, Hazel maintains that at the time of their marriage (which she says pointedly was not in a church), she did not really know how important her new husband was. Any ignorance on this count must have been quickly dispelled by a letter dated 21st. June 1950 from Arthur Condry, one of the Dental Board members. Condry wrote, "My Dear Chairman, I do sincerely wish you and your future wife every possible happiness as well as, I am sure, all your many friends who hold you not only in high esteem for your great abilities and well earned eminence but above all in affection and regard. She may not fully realise the greatness, second to none, which you have achieved in your profession and how highly you are regarded by all who know you personally." The marriage proved to be a successful partnership for the rest of Fish's life.

In the General Election of 1950 Labour was returned with a fragile majority. Food rationing had been maintained under the stringent economic reign of the Chancellor, Sir Stafford Cripps, and the following year was to see the government defeated at the polls. On April 23rd.1951, Aneurin Bevan had announced to the House of Commons his resignation as Minister of Health. Charges for teeth and spectacles as well as differences over foreign policy had been too much for Bevan to tolerate. Cripps had proposed a £13 million cut in the NHS budget, and had decided to put a ceiling on health expenditure. Bevan was furious, and demanded to know where the next squeeze would be. Hospitals? Prescriptions? The Right Hon. H.A.Marquand replaced Bevan, and the BDJ commented tartly, "It may be hoped that he will be more ready than his predecessor sometimes appeared to avail himself of the advice of the profession on whose members the ultimate success of the Health Service depends."

The conditions of the Health Service had brought new pressures and regulations to dental practitioners, and the BDA realised that its obligations to its members had changed. In its editorial it asked, "how the association can best be organised to give effect to the wishes of its members and protect their legitimate interests?" Over the years this obligation to protect the interests of the dentists working within the NHS came to be the organisation's major pre-occupation. In effect it became the 'Trade Union' of those dentists working within the NHS. Private practice was not its concern. The interests of the Dental Board were quite different.

At the 1951 General Election, although the Labour Party had actually won most votes, Churchill was back in office with a workable majority, and in that year Fish presented his eighth Chairman's Address. After congratulating W. Kelsey Fry on his knighthood, Fish proceeded to announce with satisfaction the news that in the five years since the war the number of disciplinary cases had been much lower than the number in the five years prior to the war, but the gist of his Address centred on the move of the profession to independence. He acknowledged the very cordial relations that the Board had maintained with the GMC, but said, "it has been abundantly clear that the Act of 1921 is out of date." The NHS had "placed upon the dental profession responsibilities which more than ever require that it should be a self-governing profession, responsible for its own standards of education, its own regulation and its own discipline. It follows therefore that to discharge these additional responsibilities provision must be made for a "General Dental Council" on which the profession is more widely represented..."

He went on to talk about another of his favourite topics, dental education, and announced that a small committee had been set up to look at the use of visual aids in both dental health education and education for undergraduate and postgraduate students. Thirteen films were already made for circulation to dental schools.

Fish took another opportunity to talk about education when he was given the rare honour of being elected to an Honorary Membership of the BDA. On such occasions the recipient of the award did not usually give a talk, but Fish could not be deterred from giving a rather extended address. He spoke about the advances over the years to make dentistry an academic discipline and said with pride that now every university in the country had a dental school and at least one professor of dental surgery.

Most dentists had now become relatively affluent members of the community. Through hard work over long hours, many of them were earning more than their medical colleagues, and dental schools had two-and-a-half times more applicants than available places. Fish noted that earnings were so good that final year students in Commonwealth countries book passages to England before they qualify, and that one such graduate had somehow earned £28,000 in one year.

The obvious imbalance between the demand for dental treatment and the number of dentists prompted the Teviot Committee to look to alternative ways of meeting the nation's needs. A central question was whether the necessary increased workforce should be composed of more dentists or more ancillary workers. An experiment was suggested in which a class of ancillaries similar to the New Zealand Dental Nurses, would be trained to perform extractions and fillings. The Board objected that this would break the monopoly the profession had possessed for thirty years, saying that the way forward was to train more dentists, and the Teviot Committee even proposed a shortened undergraduate curriculum "compatible with the maintenance of a satisfactory standard of training." Another proposal was the formation of a 'Civilian Dental Service', essentially a full-time salaried service with emphasis on treatment for children, an increasing need as the school dental service diminished. The salaries offered by Local Authorities could not compare with what dentists were earning in NHS practice. The BDA again put forward the idea of a grant-in-aid system which would allow dentists to be rewarded by the patient for better quality work. However much to Fish's frustration the Teviot Committee was slow to come to any decision.

Parliament was now considering the Dentists Bill 1951 which proposed to give self-government to the dental profession by establishing a General Dental Council, "whose general concern …will be…to promote high standards of professional education and conduct." This was to be an enlarged Council with a changed relationship with the GMC, in that it would not send 'additional members' to the GMC, but would now have six members of the GMC among its membership. This was far short of complete independence let alone autonomy, but it was a considerable acknowledgement of dentistry as an independent profession capable of establishing and monitoring its own standards. Fish anticipated the change with enthusiasm and increasing frustration; even by the end of 1952 the Bill had not gone beyond its first reading.

However Fish was fully occupied with other matters. He published an important paper on 'A new principle in practical denture design', which described partial dentures incorporating the principles of splint design so that teeth, especially those weakened by loss of supporting tissue, would be protected from lateral stress. This meant that the plate covered occlusal and lingual surfaces of teeth and coverage of the 'saddle areas' and gum margins could be reduced. Today we take this kind of design for granted, but then it represented a considerable innovation. As testimony to Fish's work, models are kept at the museum of the Royal College of Surgeons.

Soon after the war the Federation Dentaire Internationale (FDI) had been re-constituted, and one of its first intentions was to establish an international dental journal. This had been discussed for some years before the war, and in 1938 a draft contract had been drawn up between the FDI and the German publishers Aesculap-Verlag. Fish had been impatient to get this off the ground, but the Germans objected because Aesculap-Verlag was a Jewish firm whose business had been transferred to London. The Editorial Committee took a vote resulting in five for going ahead, the German against and the Swiss member abstaining. The Italian member who had been warned that his future in Fascist Italy now allied to Germany, would be prejudiced, nevertheless voted for the agreement. However the war intervened, and the project was dropped until after the war when the new liaison officer of the FDI and secretary of the London Congress Organising Committee, Gerald Leatherman, a London practitioner of South African origin, negotiated publishing with the London house of Cassells.

The first meeting of the editorial board of the journal was held in Fish's house at 34 Weymouth Street in the evening of the 14th. October 1948, but most subsequent meetings were held at Leatherman's address in Devonshire Place. Professor H.H. Stones from Liverpool, with whom Fish had qualified, was in the Chair and subsequently appointed editor of the new International Dental Journal. One of the first plans for the journal was to be able to report the forthcoming XI th. Dental Congress of 1952 in four languages, English, French, German and Spanish. They decided on 16 divisions of dentistry, which meant 64 components of the journal, and Cassels agreed to supply 24 tons of paper to produce 10,000 copies per quarter, each of 156 pages. Sub-editors in Dutch, Danish, French, German, Italian and Spanish were appointed. There were complaints from the French that a Belgian had been appointed to do the French translation, and a Frenchman was appointed.

Perhaps the most exotic of these people was Dr. J. Schermant, the Spanish sub-editor, dentist to the king of Spain and a friend of Fish. Schermant was born in Warsaw and became a student of Gottlieb's. During the First War he was captured by the Russians and imprisoned in Siberia, from where he escaped to China and then to the USA. He obtained a DDS at Pennsylvania Dental School. He met Fish at an FDI conference where they became good friends. He introduced Fish to modern ideas on inlays and fixed bridgework, including that great challenge to the enterprising dentist, the three-quarter crown.

After notice of its forthcoming appearance had been published in every national dental journal, the first issue of the International Dental Journal came out in September 1950; at the meeting of the Editorial Board to discuss the first issue the French correspondent complained that his report should have been longer. By 1952 the journal had over 1,500 subscribers, but Cassels reported that they were making a loss due to the late arrival of material. Not all the correspondents were as efficient as Fish.

In commenting on the role of the new journal in facilitating international exchange of thought, the spread of education, and progress to the universal provision of dental care, he said, "Slowly but inexorably universal education is abolishing privilege, and benefits which have been achieved by the once privileged classes of society are now demanded by all." Fish's father, the Wesleyan Minister, would have said no different.

Fish's major preoccupation at this time was his Presidency of the XIth. International Dental Congress held in London in the Royal Festival Hall in the new South Bank complex by the Thames, where the Festival of Britain had taken place.

The XIth. International Congress was the culmination of four years planning by the Organising Committee of which Fish was the Chairman, G.H. Leatherman the honorary secretary, A.C.R.McLeod the honorary treasurer. W.Stewart Ross, Fish's friend and partner in practice, was responsible for organising the scientific programme.

The conference was attended by 3,940 people from 26 countries, 758 from the USA. Simultaneous language interpretation was used for the first time, speakers in English, French, Spanish, Italian and German being translated into English and French. On arrival at the Festival Hall each morning delegates were given copies of the newsheet Congress Courier with up-to-date information about congress proceedings and social events.

The ceremony was opened by the Minister of Health, the Right Honourable Ian Macloed MP, and the Bishop of Southwark started the meeting with prayers. Then Fish was inducted into the Chair "accompanied by loud applause from the delegates."

In his Presidential address Fish said that a professional career called for constant refreshment of the mind, and that every person at the Congress was at heart a student. Dr. Balint Orban, a great histologist and formerly one of Gottlieb's students, now settled in the USA, was awarded the Miller prize, and Sir Alexander Fleming opened the scientific programme. A very popular innovation was the introduction of Brains Trusts when eminent members spoke informally and were questioned by the audience about their subject. There were organised visits to dental schools, cocktail parties, and a Congress Ball held in the Royal Albert Hall. A cultural tone was added when the London Philarmonic Orchestra gave a concert in honour of the Congress, and the famous violinist Alfredo Campoli played Tchaikovsky's Violin Concerto in D. A Congress Banquet was held at the Grosvenor House presided over by Fish, at which Miss Florence Horsburgh, Minister of Education, was the guest of honour.

The Congress was reckoned by all to be a huge success; it provided all those involved, delegates and the organisers in the FDI a spur to the future. For Fish it was a triumph. Whatever success he would achieve in the following years, the XIth. International Congress represented the pinnacle of his reputation on the European dental scene. In Fish's epilogue to the Congress he said, "it is impossible to assess the extent to which our Congress has been of value," and he quoted the rousing speech by

Shakespeare's Henry V after the English victory at Agincourt, "And gentlemen in England, now a-bed, Shall think themselves accurs'd they were not here."

For the dental profession at large the Congress represented a continuation of Britain's celebration of peace, and hopefully a harbinger of continuing progress.

In March 1953, Dr. Fish received an invitation to the coronation ceremony at Westminster Abbey, where on the June 2nd. Elizabeth was crowned Queen. Mrs. Fish watched the ceremony from the television set at the Athenaeum Club, of which Fish was a member.

The Dental Bill showed no sign of making progress through parliament, but Fish remained bullish about the progress of the profession, and in his next Chairman's Address, that of 1953, he ended by quoting Seneca, "Courage leads to the stars, fear towards death" and continued, " I have no doubt of our courage or of our destination, or that in the perspective of history we need fear the moral judgement of our fellow men." Perhaps this was a morale boosting speech because events were not proceeding as well as they might. Entry to dental schools was falling, a gap was evident between the standard of training students received at the university based dental schools and the work performed under the NHS, and public awareness of the value of dental health remained low. Some people remained so poor that with charges for dentures they needed support from the National Assistance Board, something that the BDA had successfully negotiated.

The following year, Fish, as Chairman of the Dental Board, was honoured with a knighthood, and because his wife Hazel did not like the name Eric, he became Sir Wilfred. In April the BDA gave a dinner for Sir Wilfred and Lady Fish at the Grosvenor House, at which the BDA President, Mr. Edgar Houghton, said of Fish, "Whatever work he had undertaken he had performed with distinction, and his fame had justly spread throughout the world."

Also in 1954, at Alexander Fleming's request, Fish gave the first Almroth Wright memorial lecture. This was held in the lecture theatre at St. Mary's, and in his introduction Fish said, "However inappropriate it may be that I should be permitted to open this 1954 series of Almroth Wright lectures, it is most appropriate that they should be held in this lecture theatre. Not only was this Institute built for Wright and his colleagues to work in, but he took an active part in the Building of it." He went on to describe the work of the great bacteriologist whom he had known as a colleague and friend, but it is significant that it was Fish and not another colleague, or even Fleming himself, who gave this first memorial lecture. Fish's eloquence and the great care that he took with such tasks were well appreciated, and one dentist who had attended his lectures thought that if Fish had gone into the law instead of dentistry he would have made a very successful barrister.

In April of that year Fish's old chief, Colyer died, soon to be followed by the demise of Alexander Fleming. In his obituary for Sir Alexander Fleming, his friend and colleague at St. Mary's Hospital, Fish described how the flower girls of Barcelona spread the streets with blooms for Fleming to walk on, and said with great truth that " there must be very few people in any civilised country who do not owe him a debt of gratitude."

Fish gave the first Wilkinson Memorial lecture at his old school in Manchester, at which Wilkinson had been professor before moving to London to run the Eastman Dental Institute. In that address Fish raised the subject of the standard of student to be recruited to dentistry. There was a manifest need for a difference to be made between the brighter student enrolled for the degree who might go on to be a teacher, and the rest, who by taking the diploma would satisfy the minimal requirements set by the GMC. This was a theme that Fish addressed many times, and in the article, 'An Enterprise in Dental Research' of May 1958, marking the establishment of the Department of Dental Science, he spelt out the characteristics to be looked for in the potential research worker, stressing the importance of "compelling curiosity" and "tremendous enthusiasm," both of which traits he possessed in abundance.

In his next Chairman's Address Fish tackled the problem of the shortage of dentists.

Young people knew little about dental health and therefore could not view dentistry as a worthwhile career, and the cost of a dental training was prohibitive to many. So far as the latter situation was concerned he recommended the revival of the Board's former bursary scheme which had been discontinued at the outbreak of war.

In an attempt to improve public awareness of the value of oral hygiene and dental health the Dental Board held a reception for the Press at which the latter expressed surprise that "on a matter so vital to public health the initiative should have been left entirely to the Board", and that the cost of all dental propaganda should be paid for out of the registration fees of the dentists. Fish called for a national campaign against "the widespread ignorance which exists in this country today on questions of oral hygiene and dental health." The cost of such a campaign was reckoned to be about a million pounds and well beyond the resources of the Board.

The Department of Health seems to have taken no part in helping with these problems. Dentistry needed to look after its own house, and one encouraging move on the part of the dental schools was the introduction of visits by sixth formers to stimulate their interest in dentistry as a worthwhile career.

At the 1954 Annual Conference of Executive Councils the Minister of Health, Ian MacLeod, declared, "my personal relationship and those of my Ministry with the dental profession are closer and friendlier than ever before" a statement which gave hope that movement on the new Dentists Act could be expected, but in his introduction to the 69th. Session of the Dental Board in 1955, Fish with wry humour masking his disappointment at the speed with which parliament was dealing with the governance of dentistry said, "We meet once more in the shadow of impending dissolution. A Bill to amend the Dentists Acts is again before Parliament and if it survives this time we shall, as a Board, pass out of existence - peacefully I trust."

Until this time the GMC had a Special Committee on the Dental Curriculum, and had a powerful voice in dental education, especially on pre-clinical subjects, and Fish referred to this when he said, "this administrative independence which is to be accorded to dentistry will not cause us to sever our connection with our friends and advisors of the General Medical Council who will continue to give the General Dental Council the benefit of their advice on all educational matters"

A major concern of the government was the shortage of dentists, and the recent 10% reduction in dental remuneration had not helped that situation. An Interdepartmental Committee under the Chairmanship of Sir Arnold McNair had been set up to look into the matter. This was another sign of the recognition that dental health mattered, and that this could not simply be left to the dental profession itself. The profession through the Dental Board had been responsible not only for keeping the Register but also for maintaining the numbers in the profession, and despite the initial increase in the numbers after the introduction of the NHS, numbers had been falling. The McNair Committee set as an objective an increase of 2-3,000 more dentists over the next ten years. Fortunately, by the time this recommendation was pronounced dental student numbers had risen and the dental schools were full. This was due to the efforts of the Board. Fish had also been able to announce the creation of 'Dental Board Scholarships' to the value of £200 per year for the length of time of the dental course up to a maximum of five years. The Board was now publishing an illustrated booklet about a career in dentistry, distributed free to schools and Local Education Authorities, and later Fish was pleased to announce that a new book on dental health was selling at a hundred copies a month.

At the last meeting of the Dental Board Fish paid tribute to Sir Francis Dyke Acland, who although not a dentist, had been given by the Privy Council the task of bringing the Dental Board into being and establishing it on a firm footing. Also Fish congratulated Fred Ballard, the long serving treasurer of the Board, on his well deserved OBE. Ballard was a '1921' man, and it must have been especially gratifying to him to see the labours of the Board, which he had served tirelessly for almost twenty years, coming to fruition in the long awaited establishment of the General Dental Council.

Chapter 13

THE GENERAL DENTAL COUNCIL

The Royal Assent to the Dentists Act 1956 was given on March15th, and it came into law on the 4th. July, thirty-five years after the Dental Board had been brought into being. The new General Dental Council was increased to 37 members, 11 of which had to be elected from the Register of Dentists. There was an immediate protest that in disciplinary cases the accused would be faced by 37 people, the majority of whom were not practising dentists. However it was pointed out that the Disciplinary Committee of the GDC was composed of only ten people with an adequate representation of practitioners as their number had been increased from three to four, and that of the remaining six members two must be laymen.

One of the most vigorously argued amendments to the Bill related to the supervision of ancillary workers. Initially the Bill had insisted that the ancillary work be under the direct supervision of the dentist. This obligation to direct supervision was modified to place a clear obligation upon the dentist to prescribe the treatment that the ancillary shall carry out. The profession did not give its support to the suggestion that ancillaries could extract deciduous teeth, or that dental technicians could work as prosthetists.

The Chairman of the Dental Board had been a Privy Council appointment, but under the Dentists Act 1957, the President of the General Dental Council was elected by the members, and Fish was duly appointed. From then on, the Privy Council had, and has, no input in the election of the President. Its sole function in relation to the Council's membership is in the appointment of the lay members.

At the first meeting of the General Dental Council on July 4th 1956, Fish spelt out its responsibilities to a self-governing profession; the control over entry and the right to expel, and the responsibilities for visiting and inspecting places of dental education, as well as the supervision of examinations. The editorial in the BDJ described medicine and dentistry as collateral professions.

Change was in the air, and what was most in evidence was the realisation that in maintaining the nation's health, including dental health, the government had further obligations. From its inception the Dental Board had had the responsibility to maintain an adequate supply of dentists. Now there was a government Committee on the Recruitment to the Dental Profession under the Chairmanship of the recently ennobled Lord McNair, which set an objective of recruiting two to three thousand more dentists over the next ten years. By happy coincidence the dental schools were now full, partly the result of the Board's success in its public relations campaigns with booklets going to schools, and the availability of scholarships. Young people were getting to know more about the potential of a career in dentistry, and at that time earnings were still relatively high. McNair confirmed that the best way to get recruits was to make the public aware of the benefits of dental health, and it looked at the possibility of making a film which "might even necessitate it being made at public expense." At that time this represented a radical change in thinking about State responsibility.

In planning the details of the National Health Service the Department of Health had studied the pre-war working practices of doctors and dentists together with their earnings, and with some idea of the future demand for health services worked out a system of remuneration under the Service. So far as dentists were concerned the calculations had been wildly off the mark. Demand was vastly greater than anticipated, and dentists prepared to work much longer hours. An Interdepartmental Committee on the Remuneration of General Dental Practitioners was set up under the Chairmanship of Sir Will Spens to decide on what might be a reasonable range of professional earnings for a dentist working not more than 1500 chair-side hours per year, with the notion that a dentist should have an annual income of £1,600 in terms of 1939 values, that is somewhat less than a doctor might earn but comfortable none the less. However it was much less than many earned in private practice.

In 1957 at the fifth session of the Council, Fish announced progress in the planning of a class of ancillaries, the dental hygienists. The role of regular scaling and instruction in oral hygiene instruction in disease prevention had long been recognised; it was one of Fish's hobby-horses, and prevention formed the main theme of Fish's Presidential Address to the Royal Society of Health's Section of Preventive Medicine. As ever the sweep of his talk was wide, and in reviewing the history of preventive medicine's role in prolonging life, he cited the problem of Japan's ever increasing population. National resources were strained and the size of the population a threat to the standard of living, so abortion was legalised. For each live birth at least one pregnancy was terminated surgically. Fish commented that, "Not only is this remedy more hateful than nature's own law (miscarriage), but the end-result is devoid of the redeeming feature of natural selection."

In describing Britain's comparative position in fighting dental disease he pointed out that Britain's dentist to population ratio was 1: 3,273, Norway 1:2,000 and the USA 1:1,667 . We had six and a half million children and three and a half million mothers in need of dental care. The urgent need to reduce disease prevalence demanded advice on oral hygiene and the addition of fluoride to drinking water. Further it needed Treasury support for dental care campaigns.

Despite his heavy commitment to dental politics, probably as a welcome counterpoint, Fish still had time and energy to give a demonstration in the radiography department at St. Mary's Hospital on tongue space for dentures, a matter he considered to be very important in denture design and stability. He did this by radiographing dentures painted with radiopaque paint, or by pouring plaster of Paris between articulated dentures and demonstrating the limited space for the tongue.

It was no longer the responsibility of Council to help in the building of dental schools, but Council did have other educational programmes under way. Although progress on organising a programme of training for hygienists was slow, the

Ancillary Workers Curriculum Sub-Committee under the vigorous chairmanship of Robert Bradlaw was making progress on what was called the Ancillary Workers Experimental Scheme. This scheme, which was proposed in the Dental Act, and for which government money had been approved in 1957, was to introduce a class of ancillaries modelled on the New Zealand Dental Nurse programme, that is where after a two-year course people, usually young ladies, were qualified to carry out extraction of deciduous teeth, perform simple fillings and scalings. A site on the grounds of New Cross Hospital had been allocated for the buildings. The building agreement was signed two years later.

In 1958 Fish was re-elected as Dean of the Faculty of Dental Surgery of the Royal College of Surgeons of England, and Sir Charles Wheeler, President of the Royal Academy of Arts gave a talk on the Dentist as Artist. What better accolade could there be for a profession once regarded as a bunch of rogues and butchers.

The following year brought the re-election of Fish as Council President for another five years. The various committees and their chairmen were appointed. Fish was on four committees and chairman of two, the Disciplinary Committee and the Preliminary Proceedings Committee. Bradlaw was on eight committees including the Education Committee. As the first Dean of the Faculty of Dental Surgery of the Royal College of Surgeons of England, and a member of the Teviot Committee he possessed a powerful voice, especially in matters of dental education and negotiations with the Ministry of Health. Dr. W.G. Senior, the Principal Dental Officer at the Ministry of Health was on seven committees, Sir W. Kelsey Fry and Professor M.A. Rushton, both from Guy's, and Professor Roberts, Dean of the Sheffield school, were on three, and other members were on one or two. This included the newly appointed Dean at Leeds, and one of Bradlaw's former staff at Newcastle, Professor Fred Hopper. It was easy to see where power and influence lay. Ballard, one of the oldest members, was on nine committees and continued to be Honorary Treasurer. The academics on Council recognised where a business head was needed.

In that year Fish gave one of his most quoted talks, entitled 'A Profession In The Making'. In effect it was a call to arms, in which he described the advances and setbacks in the history of dentistry, finishing with the words, " It would be contrary to all human experience to suppose that any single event, however momentous, could change the whole course of history without further continuing effort." When the Council met for the first time in its own Council Chamber in the new building on Wimpole Street, this made, as Fish said, "the final expression of that independence which was granted to the dental profession three years ago."

In that year he was appointed Honorary Consultant in Dental Surgery to the Army. This honour was soon followed by Fish receiving an Honorary Fellowship of the Royal Microscopical Society in recognition of his pioneer work in dental pathology.

Two matters of great concern came up at the next meeting of Council. These were 1) to provide some scheme for the dental care of children, and 2) the need to recruit and train graduates capable of teaching and carrying out research in prevention of disease.

Fish said that it was much to the credit of the profession that of the 16,000 dentists a thousand are found with the altruism to make either a part-time or full-time contribution to the school dental service.

He was very pleased to be able to describe the gracious visit of the Duke of Edinburgh and the Minister of Health, Enoch Powell, to the Council's new premises for the formal opening on the 9th November 1960, and also the fact that the first entry of sixty young women to the new School for Dental Auxiliaries at New Cross had taken place. At the opening ceremony of the new training school on the 19th.December 1960, Enoch Powell, in introducing the subject of dental health said, "Nature, for some inscrutable reason has decreed that the human race shall find the subject of dental pain and its relief exquisitely amusing - to everyone except the parties concerned." A psychologist could have explained to the Minister that laughter and fear are close colleagues, but the statement did reflect contemporary attitudes to dentistry, a subject of great concern to Fish. The image of the profession as well matters of professional conduct occupied regular space in his annual addresses. The names and addresses, even photographs, of some dentists had appeared in the Press, and although this was often connected with articles on dentistry, in some cases this represented undesirable publicity and advertising for material advantage. Fish deplored lapses of this kind, even when the dentist in question had instructed a journalist not to disclose his identity, that was not enough, except in special cases of public interest.

Even more disturbing was the decision by the Judicial Council of the Privy Council to overturn a decision of the Disciplinary Committee. This committee had found a dentist guilty of infamous and disgraceful conduct and erased his name from the Register. It seems that the culprit claimed fees for fillings he had not carried out. He blamed this wrongful claim on secretarial carelessness, but the Disciplinary Committee took the view that he had acted dishonestly, fraudulently and recklessly.

The Judicial Council of the Privy Council took the view that the extreme professional penalty of erasure from the Register was justified in cases of moral turpitude or fraud and reckless disregard of the dentist's duty concerning records, and of these the accused was not guilty. It was an admonition to the Council to be more careful.

Certainly the Council at that time did seem to overact in what it perceived as unprofessional conduct. Too large a brass name plate could elicit a complaint, and in advertising for staff, dentists must not put their name or address in the newspaper, but could put their telephone number rather than a box number which had been the original strictly enforced requirement.

Another concern was the patient complaint that dentists refused to carry out certain work except privately. This infringed NHS regulations, but given the scale of fees for more advanced work many on the Council, who had been in favour of a grant-in-aid system of payment, must have been sympathetic to dentists involved.

On the 14th. November of 1963 such a case appeared before

the disciplinary committee with Fish in the Chair. John Denis Moore, who practised on the East India Dock Road, London, was charged with persuading Mrs. J. Paterson to undergo a certain course of dental treatment as a private patient by falsely stating that such treatment was not available under the National Health Service. That course of treatment was periodontal, for which Mr. Moore demanded £20 of which the patient paid £8. Mr. Moore was found "guilty of infamous or disgraceful conduct in a professional respect" and his name was erased from the Register.

Mr. Moore appealed and the case went before the Judiciary Committee of the Privy Council. They took the view that the charge against Moore was in effect of obtaining money from a patient by false pretences. The appellant's case was that the patient had pyorrhoea which needed treatment, that he was qualified (by dint of studying this in America) to do so, but that it could not be done under the National Health Service because of the length of time it would take. It appeared that Moore had never stated that treatment could not be done *at all* under the NHS, but that he could not do it because the NHS would not stand for the fee. The crux of the matter, as Their Lordships saw it, was whether at the Disciplinary Committee of the GDC Moore had been asked by anyone whether he had actually said to the patient that periodontal treatment was not available under the Health Service, or just that he could not do it. There was doubt, and Their Lordships came to the conclusion that Moore's answers to the Committee's questions had been equivocal. For that reason they allowed the appeal and Moore's name was restored to the Register. The costs of the appellant had to be paid by the respondent, the GDC. The actions of the disciplinary committee against these dentists may well have been dictated by Fish's own standards of ethical behaviour. It is possible that with his long-standing authority, Fish was able to impose his own strict Wesleyan code of conduct to what he saw as unprofessional behavious to bear on the committee's decision. He was then approaching seventy, and possibly becoming something of a martinet.

By 1962, the year in which fifty Dental Auxiliary students

qualified, to be employed by enthusiastic Local Education Authorities, Fish was involved in a larger arena of activity. The Council was considering the problems associated with the entry of Britain into the European Economic Community, which required harmonising standards of professional qualifications.

Matters of education were the subject of the Evelyn Sprawson Lecture which Fish gave at the London Hospital Medical College on the 16th. February 1963. It was a classic Fish presentation in which he brought Pythagoras, Plato and Bacon to his aid in describing the liberalisation of specialist education and the training of graduates for teaching and research. In many ways it was his farewell address to his profession, for he retired from the Council in the following year. The last act of homage from his profession while Fish was still on the Council, was the award of the Colyer Gold Medal of the Royal College of Surgeons of England for "one who has done so much for dental surgery and the advancement of dental research."

On the 4th July 1964 Bradlaw followed Fish as President of the Council, and in one of many tributes paid at that meeting, quoted Edmund Burke that " great men are both landmarks and guideposts. Sir Wilfred is such a man; it has been given to few to weave the fabric of dental history as he has done." Referring to Fish's radical examination of many former common practices, Bradlaw said, "too often orthodoxy is celibate", and he then went on to quote Carlyle, who defined statesmanship as the ability to foresee the needs of those who come after us. "This Sir Wilfred has done. He has given us firm foundation on which to build the future of our profession."

Fish was deeply moved. In his many years on the Dental Board and then on the Council, twenty years in the Chair, he had had to announce the passing of so many friends and colleagues, and he replied that he was happy to have been invited to be present. Had he not been invited he would have been present in spirit, but he was much happier to be present in the flesh.

Chapter 14

THE FACULTY OF DENTAL SURGERY

In May 1938 the Board of Examiners in Dental Surgery at the Royal College of Surgeons of England considered the desirability of the College instituting a post-graduate diploma in Dental Surgery. They felt that such a diploma would be in the interests of the dental health of the community as well as being advantageous to those who obtained it. The title Higher Diploma (HDDS,RCS) was considered, but under the existing charter of the College, a higher diploma was not permissible.

In July 1939 the higher diploma was further discussed, and the title Master Surgeon Dentist (MSD,RCS, Eng) was suggested. It was then resolved that a petition be submitted for a supplementary charter to give the College power to grant a higher diploma, but the war intervened.

On the night of 10/11 May 1941 three high explosive bombs fell directly on the College and caused tremendous destruction. The damage even extended to the sub-basement destroying part of the Hunterian collection of specimens stored there. What remained of the College building was an uninhabitable shell, but the President, Sir Alfred Webb-Johnson brought immense drive not only to the rebuilding, but to ideas about the future purpose of the College. He envisaged the College as a centre of medical sciences, and was keen to keep the activity of the newly emerging surgical specialities within the College umbrella. It is said that during an air raid in 1941 Webb-Johnson and Sir Henry Souttar, distinguished surgeon and Vice-President of the College, discussed the formation of specialist Faculties within the College, an idea which enjoyed general support and brought the Faculty of Dental Surgery into being.

The year 1942 saw a new department of ophthalmic research, the foundation of new Chairs in Pathology and Anatomy, and attention was given to the further development of off-site centres. One of these was at East Grinstead Hospital where Archibald

McIndoe was making revolutionary strides in plastic surgery, particularly in the treatment of burns, and where Kelsey Fry had established the foremost maxillo-facial surgery unit.

Anaesthesia and dental surgery were prominent in these plans, and the matter of the higher dental diploma came up again in May 1943 when a memorandum about the diploma was submitted to the Council. A year later an Extraordinary Meeting of the Council of the College under the Chairmanship of Webb-Johnson, was held to read the memorandum. It was resolved that the resolution of 1939 be confirmed, with the exception of the title, and that leading dental surgeons be consulted in regard to the diploma being entitled Fellow in Dental Surgery (FDSRCS, Eng.). At the same meeting the Council considered granting higher diplomas in other special branches of surgery, such as Ophthalmology.

At about this time the pressing need for establishing dentistry on a firm scientific foundation, which had been recognised by Fish and many others for years, took on some reality.

In Fish's notes he recalls the following conversation.

" 'Could you spend a million pounds on dentistry?' That question was put to me by Lord Bracken when he was Minister of Information during the war." Fish wrote about this time. "He had come to see me professionally and as often happened stayed to have a talk for a few minutes. Naturally I said 'Yes' but was quickly overtaken (and overcome) by the question, 'How?' .I therefore said that I would spend the money training teachers to a standard comparable with that of other university disciplines.

Brendan Bracken's response was immediate. He slapped his knee, jumped up and started towards the door . 'Train teachers', he said, 'that's it.' 'Yes,' I said, 'but just wait a minute. How will you get the million pounds?' I can still see the wicked look he gave me over his shoulder saying, 'Give someone a peerage for it' - and was gone."

Training teachers and dental research workers was a theme that had occupied Fish's thoughts and writing for many years, and had formed a regular topic of discussion with Professor Lovatt Evans, in whose department at UCL Fish carried out the research for which he was awarded his D.Sc.

The Nuffield Foundation was founded during the war in June 1943, and by then Nuffield was already a peer of many years standing, and through the Nuffield Trust a notable supporter of health care institutions. It was a time when with a dentist: population ratio of 1:5,000, the need for more dentists had become urgent. There was an even worse shortage of dental teachers as most were in the Services. Fish reports that there were only thirty in all sixteen dental schools put together. The student numbers were down, but Fish predicted that there would be a post-war rush as there had been in 1919. Recruitment was a problem that had worried him since he had been elected to the Dental Board of the United Kingdom.

At a meeting of the Trustees of the Nuffield Foundation, which was held at the Savoy Hotel on the 22nd. July 1944, one of the items on the agenda was to consider which areas of medical research to support. Dentistry, ophthalmology, rheumatology, and research into catarrh were mentioned, for which a sum of £180,000 could be set aside. But Mr. W. Hyde, the Public Relations Officer, stated that while Lord Nuffield hoped that these four items could receive attention, this was not quite what he had in mind. He considered that dentistry was the most important item with ophthalmology next, and that a Chair in Dentistry should be set up without delay, he hoped at Oxford.

At the next meeting of the trustees they had before them three memoranda, one from "Dr.E.W.Fish and Mr. Alfred E. Rowlett on the present state and prospects of dental education and research," another from Kelsey Fry on the establishment of a Chair in Dental Health, and a further one from Fish on training for an academic career in dentistry, for both education and research.

The trustees came to the conclusion there that was urgent need for stimulating research, for increasing the number of dentists and improving their quality. It was agreed that a small advisory committee should be set up to advise the trustees.

A week or two later Fish was invited to attend a meeting of this Advisory Committee on Dentistry which consisted of five eminent medical academics, of whom, as Fish was very pleased to find, Lovatt Evans was one, to discuss his memoranda.

"When to my surprise and delight I received a letter from the Foundation asking when could they receive my proposals for training dental teachers," Fish wondered whether his conversation with Brendan Bracken had anything to do with it, but he felt sure that earlier discussions with Lovatt Evans were significant. Some time before the Nuffield Scheme was started Lovatt Evans had said to Fish, " Send me a few of your best students. I will show them how to do research - not on dental problems - possibly on the glycogen content of heart muscle - but when I have finished with them they will be able to tackle any problem - dental or otherwise."

The terms of reference of the advisory committee were to advise on the ways in which the Foundation could help most effectively the improvement in dental education in Great Britain, and the necessary research in physiology, biochemistry and pathology.

Subsequently the Advisory Committee on Dentistry had several meetings, and on the 5th. October 1944 at the trustees' meeting, the matter of Scholarships and Fellowships in various subjects, including dentistry, was one of the main items on the agenda. By this time the committee had invited the opinion of other experts including Dr. Weaver of the Board of Education, and Lady Mellanby, who replied that she felt unable to be of any great help in the discussions.

In his submissions Fish had emphasised the need to provide Scholarships for brilliant students to enable them to take a B.Sc degree before completing their dental training, and to provide Fellowships for graduates to pursue research in dentistry, medicine or science, with perhaps a Ph.D. at the end of it.

One of the central considerations of the trustees concerned the limits of its function, that is where a line should be drawn beyond which support for teaching and research institutions should be the responsibility of the government. This corresponded with the concern of the Dental Board. The dental profession itself, through the Dental Board had funded dental schools and dental training, and apart from the school clinics which were the province of the Local Education Authority, almost every other aspect of dental health. Fish's years at the Board had convinced him of both the injustice and the uncertainty of such responsibility. Very gradually politicians had come to realise that the responsibility for certain aspects of the nation's life, in particular health and education, could not be supported by the precarious whim of charity, or by vested interests, but must be the responsibility of the community at large, that is of the government. Where did this leave research?

Fish realised that before the support of any official bodies, such as Local Education Authorities, could be recruited, any project that he had in mind would be viewed as experimental until it had proved its worth in practise. Therefore garnering funds from private bodies, industry and commerce, was essential. The Nuffield Foundation, reflecting Lord Nuffield's own strongly held beliefs, was at that time, along with the Rowntree Trust, among the most far-sighted and benevolent of all such organisations, and its Advisory Committee on Dentistry did not disappoint Fish.

If one needed any further evidence that Fish was a driving force for change it lies in his negotiations with the Nuffield Foundation. He brought to this task his energy and his eloquence in discussion and in drafting letters and memoranda. Also, and equally important if not more so, he brought to those personal contacts, whose understanding and assistance were required, his enthusiasm for the importance of the project.

The Advisory Committee made a great number of recommendations, but stated explicitly that funding dental schools, now recognised as academic institutions, undergraduate and postgraduate training, and the training of teachers, was a matter for the Teviot Committee and the government.

Its first recommendation that a Chair in Dental Health be set up in Oxford, was certainly a sop to Lord Nuffield, and its second recommendation that the Chair be in a provincial university recognised reality. The committee report says of the status of dentistry, " the dental profession is suffering from an inferiority complex and its members are not accorded the same standing by the general public as are those of other learned professions.... a Chair of Dentistry at either Oxford or Cambridge would tend to raise the status of the profession and encourage both teaching and research."

The reasons given for the difficulties involved in promoting this idea are revealing. The report said, "It is not advisable for the following reasons:

- There is no dental school at either university and no dental hospital in either city.
- Neither Oxford nor Cambridge gives a degree or diploma in dentistry, and
- There is no indication that either university would welcome the establishment within it of a dental school."

The source of any inferiority complex was not far to seek. However the committee did suggest that Oxford and Cambridge should be asked to consider granting a degree in dentistry. Of course nothing came of it, and Fish the graduate of a 'red brick' university, cannot have expected otherwise, especially remembering his encounters with the Mellanbys.

The committee stated that its support be confined to funding fundamental research and financing a dental research institution in a dental school attached to a university, and it went on to describe the necessary personnel and their terms of employment. It recommended scholarships and bursaries of £200-300 per year to support promising students to prepare for research activity, and fellowships for graduates in dentistry and of pure science subjects such as biochemistry, to go into research and teaching.

Physiology and pathology figured large in their thinking, and it is likely that Fish's emphasis on these subjects, with the support of Lovatt Evans, distinguished physiologist, carried weight in this direction. It is also possible that Fish's influence manifested itself in their recommendation that departments of oral hygiene be instituted in all voluntary hospitals.

They estimated that the financial commitment over ten years amounted to £30,000 for scholarships and fellowships, £50,000 for a research centre, and £120,000 to university departments for improved teaching and research; a grand total of £200,000.

At further meetings these recommendations received some modifications and additions, such as funding a study of dental health in other *civilised* countries (a study of dental conditions in *uncivilised* countries would be valuable but not feasible at this time), but the substance of the committee's reports to the trustees remained the same.

At their eleventh meeting in July 1945 the Advisory Committee received further memoranda from Bradlaw, Fish, Kelsey Fry and Wilkinson on a working plan for "an ideal university department of dentistry," that is where the best teaching and research would be carried out. It is not surprising that three of the four schools considered for support were Newcastle, Guy's and Manchester; the fourth being Leeds where Professor Matthew Stewart, a member of the Advisory Committee, was Dean of the Medical School. By this time Fish no longer had a connection with a dental school. Detailed memoranda were submitted by Bradlaw for Newcastle, Wilkinson for Manchester, where a department of preventive dentistry was proposed; by Professor T. Talmage Read, Dean of the Dental School at Leeds, and significantly by the Dean of Guy's Medical School on behalf of the Dental School. The grants to these four schools over ten years were £25,000, £30,000, £10,000 and £25,000 respectively, the Leeds plan for one research worker being the most modest. The RDH, UCH Dental School, and the schools at Birmingham, Liverpool and Sheffield are not mentioned at all.

By January 1946 confirmation of these decisions had been made by the Trust, and two Fellowships were established, for D.J.Anderson to obtain a B.Sc. and possibly then an M.Sc., and for Major W.R.Roberts to obtain a medical degree. A grant-in-aid of £200 for one year was made to C.V.Smith to enable him to teach dental mechanics. The Nuffield Foundation's projects for dentistry were up and running.

Anderson was to become a professor at Guy's, and Roberts a Consultant Dental Surgeon in Birmingham. A third Fellow of 1946, A.S.Prophet, who was supported in his studies in physiology and bacteriology, was to become the Dean of UCH Dental School and then Dean of the Medical School.

By the end of the war plans for a Faculty of Dental Surgery and its Fellowship were well under way, and Bradlaw was to be a considerable influence in both. He with Colyer, Sprawson and Stobie, were dental members of the John Tomes Prize Committee.

He was the youngest member, and in his eight years as Director of Dental Studies at Newcastle had shown himself to be a dynamic and effective administrator. He was also the Chairman of the Examiners for the LDS RCS, therefore it is not surprising that as a representative of Dental Surgery he was invited to attend Council meetings to discuss the implementation of the Fellowship. By 1945 the title had been approved and regulations for obtaining a fellowship drafted. The first regulation stated that a medical qualification was not required; medicine's grip on dentistry was being relaxed. Soon after, Bradlaw was authorised to submit a memorandum on the question of establishing a Faculty of Dental Surgery at the College, and on the 31st. July 1947 the Faculty of Dental Surgery was brought into being with Bradlaw as the first Dean. By then he had resigned from the Dental Board; his workload was considerable without that responsibility.

At the first annual meeting of the Faculty on July 16th. 1948, the now Lord Webb-Johnson, as President of the College, said, " I hope and believe the creation of this Faculty will give, and indeed I feel it has already given practising dental surgeons the feeling that at long last they have a suitable academic home. Dental surgery must have its opportunity to develop not only in great hospitals but also in universities. It must have an academic home of its own, and please God as the result of the history we make together today you will find that home in the Royal College of Surgeons of England."

As Bradlaw recalled many years later, it was as a result of Webb-Johnson's vision and the subsequent invitation of a Dental Surgeon to the College Council that gave formal recognition to "Dental Surgery as a speciality of surgery on a comparable basis to Obstetrics, Ophthalmic Surgery, etc."

At the same time Bradlaw was appointed to represent the College on the Ministry of Education's panel to consider applications for awards. The BDA had played a consultative role in the institution of the Faculty, and the President of the College, the President of the BDA, Kelsey Fry, Greenish, Crook and Bradlaw were on the Fellowship regulation committee. The General Medical Council agreed that the Fellowship could be registered as an additional qualification in the Dentists Register, over which the GMC still had some say, and the first examinations were planned for February 1948. As the first Dean of the Faculty of Dental Surgery Bradlaw had to lay the foundations of the Faculty, as he said, to maintain the Hunterian tradition. Wilkinson was appointed Vice-Dean. The foundation of the Faculty coincided almost exactly with the inception of the National Health Service.

Bradlaw and Kelsey Fry were nominated to serve on perhaps the most influential of all the supervisory bodies, the Standing Dental Advisory Committee of the Ministry of Health, and in the November of 1948, Bradlaw was appointed Honorary Professor of Dental Pathology in the College. The main business of the Faculty in the next few years was largely devoted to the Fellowship examination and to postgraduate education, and both Bradlaw and Wilkinson, Deans of important dental schools, were vigorous in determining its high standard. At the invitation of the Nuffield Foundation both men made extensive tours of American dental schools to observe their methods of education. Other matters included decisions about the recognition of foreign qualifications, a matter which exercises the College to this day.

In 1950 Bradlaw resigned from the College Council, to be replaced as Dean by Kelsey Fry. Fish was elected to the Board and became Vice-Dean. In the following year Kelsey Fry, appointed CBE in 1945, was knighted.

The relationship of these two men was cordial, and although with their wives they were on visiting terms, they never seem to have established a real friendship. There may have been an element of rivalry between them. Kelsey Fry was slightly older and as a pioneer with Sir Harold Gillies in maxillo-facial surgery, not to speak of his Military Cross, his war service had been very distinguished. As a consultant to the armed forces and to the government his influence, particularly in appointments, was considerable. Both men were highly respected Dental Surgeons at prestigious hospitals, Kelsey Fry at Guy's and at East Grinstead, and Fish at St. Mary's, and both had flourishing private practices, each with a galaxy of celebrity patients. Kelsey Fry was never tempted to move into the Harley Street area, and as a Guy's man through and through, preferred to practise in a house almost next door to the hospital.

With Frank Wilkinson, who had also been part of Gillies' First World War surgical team, Kelsey Fry had been very influential in the metamorphosis of the Eastman Dental Clinic into the Postgraduate Dental Institute. He had also been a government adviser about dentistry prior to the institution of the National Health Service. The nation's honours were conferred on him just a few years earlier than on Fish. But in the political world of the Dental Board and the GDC, Fish was the more influential.

Although Bradlaw was no longer on the College Council, he was still a star in the dental firmament, and when he gave the Webb-Johnson lecture on Oral Syphilis it was, as reported in the BDJ, attended by 341 people, a larger audience than for anyone else. While Fish and others were fine lecturers, no-one then could compete with Bradlaw's charisma. As Professor 'Loma' Miles was to write many years later in Bradlaw's obituary, "He was a dental luminary of Olympian stature," and it was in no small measure due to his industry and vision that the Faculty of Dental Surgery was established.

Around this time the Board of the Faculty was giving consideration to the establishment of a Department of Dental Science.

In 1952 an Institute of Basic Medical Sciences was established at the College. It was controlled partly by the University of London through the British Postgraduate Medical Federation, and partly by the College. Within the Institute an Academic Board responsible for the organisation of postgraduate training, was set up with Bradlaw as its Chairman. Research was now in the precincts of the College, and the first idea of a Department of Dental Science was in the wind. At the same time there were plans for a Diploma in Orthodontics, and for the establishment of a hospital grade of a whole-time general dental surgeon, which was a particular concern of Wilkinson's, who in 1953 followed Kelsey Fry as Dean of the Faculty.

In 1953, Dr. W.G.Senior, the Principal Dental Officer at the Ministry of Health, and a close friend of Fish, reported that 16% of the total population of England wore full dentures, and that in the first five years of the NHS, one hundred million pounds had been spent on false teeth. In addressing a Preventive Medicine session at the Congress of the Royal Society of Health, Senior made the point that the USA had about twice as many dentists per thousand people as England (USA 1:1,700; England ,1:3,200). Thus the huge demand, taken together with a shortage of dentists, highlighted the need for more knowledge of the causes of dental disease so that preventive measures could be implemented. The establishment of a research department at the College represented the fulfilment of Fish's dream, and in 1955, the year after he was knighted, he was appointed Honorary Director of the new Department of Dental Science, and the Council of the College allocated 3,000 square feet in the rebuilt College for the department.

In July 1955 Fish gave the second Webb-Johnson Commemoration lecture. Over the years at the College, the Webb-Johnson's had become close friends of Hazel and Wilfred Fish, possibly because Manchester University was also Webb-Johnson's alma mater. Fish devoted some of the lecture to the great personalities, Rutherford prominent among them, whom Webb-Johnson and Fish had known in their student days. As always Fish took great care in the preparation of this lecture, the early drafts are numerous and fiercely edited, the final result producing an emotional letter of gratitude from Lady Webb-Johnson.

In 1956 Fish was elected Dean of the Faculty, a position he held until 1959.

Chapter 15

The British Society of Periodontology

The British Society for Periodontology was founded in 1949, the year after the first full-time department of the speciality in Britain was established at the Eastman Dental Hospital under the direction of W.G.Cross, who was probably the first specialist periodontist in the country. In 1948 when Fish received his CBE, the first edition of his book, 'Surgical Pathology of the Mouth,' came out, and by this time a reprinted and fully revised edition of his 'Parodontal Disease' had been on the market for two years. Fish's books provided a considerable impetus for British dentists to involve themselves in periodontal treatment, a subject scarcely touched on by their undergraduate training, and the teaching programmes of Cross' department were designed for those people who wished to bring themselves up-to-date. Other post-war courses in Europe were often given by American periodontists, and their message and enthusiasm subsequently transmitted to British dentists by those who taught the subject part-time at British schools. Douglas Munns, recently out of the Royal Navy was one of these. After demobilisation he became a Demonstrator for two sessions a week in the department set up at the RDH by Fish in 1932, and since 1937 officially run by the distinguished oral surgeon, Ben Fickling, after Fish left the RDH in high dudgeon at the limitations put on his research by the medical committee. Fickling had been appointed after he had accompanied Fish to Vienna for the 8th. International Dental Congress, where Gottlieb had been a prominent figure.

Munns' duties were increased to half a week when he was put in day-to-day charge of the department and responsible for undergraduate teaching. At that time Fickling's duties, like Fish's before him, consisted of a half a day a week session, occupying a dental chair at the side of the general treatment clinic. This inadequate situation was reflected at other dental schools, but gradually university demands imposed full time teaching on the ruling medical committees. However it was not until 1957 that the department at the RDH became directed by a full-time teacher, A.B.Wade, who had been a Senior Registrar at St. George's Hospital.

By 1948 every dental school in the USA had a well established periodontal department, some of them dating from the beginning of the century, and even as early as 1910, the year that Fish started his professional training, an oral hygiene department had been set up at the Forsyth Dental Infirmary in Boston, Massachusetts, where hygienists cleaned children's teeth and instructed them in oral hygiene techniques. In 1915 a hygienist school was set up in Bridport, Connecticut, and a sufficient number of American dentists took a serious interest in the subject for the American Academy of Periodontology to be founded in 1916. Even in Europe, despite the authority of the Vienna school's record on research on dental anatomy and pathology, including Gottlieb's morphological description of periodontal disease, the subject did not receive concerted interest until 1938 when The International Association for Research into Periodontal Diseases (ARPA) was formed in Frankfurt with members from many European countries. There may have been plans to form a British Society prior to World War II, but any such plans, of which there are no records, would have been delayed by the war, and it is necessary to look elsewhere to explain why Britain lagged so far behind the USA in establishing the speciality.

Concern about dental health and oral hygiene is linked with personal well-being, and with concern for personal cleanliness and hygiene in general. The individual's valuation of dental health reflects their personal feeling of worth. A good looking dentition in a healthy mouth is not only a boon in itself but represents, like clean and neat clothing, an evaluation of self, and when dental care has to be paid for it can also be regarded as a sign of relative affluence.

In the early part of the twentieth century the standard of living of the bulk of the working population in Britain was low. The industrialisation of the nineteenth century had left its mark especially on the poor, many of whom lived in squalor. Back-to-back houses had outside lavatories shared by several families, the kitchen sink was the only source of water for cooking and washing; toothbrushes were rare and often shared. In short, such were the vicissitudes of life in the conditions of poverty and ill-health at that time, that people's expectations of betterment were low. As is often cited, in the First World War only one in three conscripts was found to be fit enough to join the forces. Since the Boer War the government had realised that the efficiency of the fighting man could be compromised by dental disease, and in the 1914-18 war toothbrushes were issued to the troops. The February 1919 issue of the magazine "Brushmaking" published the obituary of the founder of the toothbrush manufacturers, Addis Ltd., in which it reported that "During the war, the firm made millions of toothbrushes for our own army and the Allied governments, all of these toothbrushes were hand drawn." In making a bone toothbrush there were over fifty separate operations.

The incidence of dental disease, both caries and periodontal disease, was so high that gum bleeding was regarded as normal, and loss of teeth inevitable and even part of the ageing process, a view shared by many dentists.

In the USA social mobility and people's expectations of life were much higher. The USA had overtaken the Europeans as the great industrial and economic power. Material success and improved social status seemed possible for those who worked hard, and the demand for dental care followed increased self-respect. The provision of dental services was also much better than in Britain. American dental training was lighter on medical science, but was more rigorous in practical and technical matters than in Britain, and produced restorative and prosthetic dentistry of such a high order that a British dentist with American training enjoyed an elevated status when he returned home. The difference between American and British dentistry can be attributed to two factors, first the drive and ready acceptance of innovation in the New World, and secondly the differences in structure and status of dentistry in the two countries.

The American dentist enjoyed autonomy from the medical

profession, the mouth was his kingdom into which he could bring all his expertise. The dentition had to be preserved, and loss of teeth, (as it was regarded in some European countries) represented failure. It followed that periodontal disease and oral hygiene received proper attention. In Britain dental schools were run by medical committees, on which sat the Honoraries, almost always doubly qualified, and this was especially the case in London where the Royal College of Surgeons set the standards. Oral surgery and prosthetics dominated the activity in their practices and their work at the dental hospitals, and therefore these two subjects were prominent on the dental school curriculum. Oral surgery put the dental surgeon on a par with colleagues in other surgical specialities, and scaling for the treatment of "gum disease" was regarded as a menial activity, certainly not one for which a medical qualification was needed. It was an activity that should be delegated to an auxiliary - if only there was such a person. The public generally were ill-informed and apathetic about dental health, and too often associated dentists only with pain. 'Blood and vulcanite' describes the panorama of British dentistry at that time, and inevitably public perception of dentistry as a profession was low. Both the public and the profession itself saw it as subordinate and inferior to medicine; the standard of entry to the profession was lower than that into medicine, a fact that deterred rather than encouraged many young people, especially the brightest, from looking to a future in dentistry. It would not be an exaggeration to say that the morale of the profession was low. This state of affairs needs to be contrasted with the situation across the Atlantic where many dentists were deeply involved with and proud of their profession. This is nowhere better exemplified than in the foundation and activity of the Pankey Institute.

L.D.Pankey graduated from the University of Louisville Dental School in 1924, and was therefore about a decade younger than Fish. Pankey's aspirations were more limited than Fish's. As Pankey said, he chose to commit his life to saving teeth. "The goal for my practice is simply to help my patients retain all their teeth all their lives if possible, in maximum comfort, function, health and aesthetics." He was a missionary for dentistry at a time when the notion of focal infection cast a shadow over much of conservative dentistry. He taught a theory of Oral Rehabilitation in which the masticatory apparatus is regarded as a functioning unit in which all parts are interdependent, a concept so far removed from the practice of dentistry in Britain as to be on a different planet. Pankey's teaching flourished, and in 1970 the L.D. Pankey Institute for Advanced Dental Education was founded to become a world-wide organisation, with members even in Britain.

Although Fish's early work and interests were not restricted to oral surgery and prosthetics, these activities formed a major part of his work. Once he had completed the research for his MD and started on his eight-year quest to clarify the physiology of the dental tissues, his first paper, read in 1924 to the Odontological Section of the RSM was on compound composite odontomes, to be followed in 1926 by an article for the RDH Review on 'Stability and Art in Full Denture Prosthesis.' Articles on Apical Infection, Pathology of Dental Caries, and Major Dental Operations on the Jaws were written many years before periodontology drew his attention. Interestingly, in the same year (1931) that he wrote an article on 'An Analysis of the Stabilising Factors in Full Denture Construction', he also gave a paper to the British Society of Orthodontics on 'Dr Gottlieb's Work on Traumatic Occlusion.'

Fish had met Gottlieb at the 8th. International Dental Congress in Vienna, and his interest in periodontal disease was provoked; the stability of dentures and tooth stability provided the linking factor.

Fortunately Fish was not the only person promoting interest in disease of the tooth-supporting tissues. For many years men like Gilmour and Sim Wallace had been preaching the role of a sound diet and good oral hygiene practice in the control of dental disease, and even as early as 1896 William Hern MRCS LDS, had a paper entitled, 'Oral Hygiene' published in the Journal of the British Dental Association. Once the Dental Board was established programmes for dental health education were instituted on a large scale. The Board had an allocated budget of £4-5,000 to carry out a programme of dental health education, and with leaflets, posters, lectures and films used the money to good effect. The tooth paste manufacturer, Messrs, D&W Gibbs and Co. set up the Ivory Castle League which was hugely successful in disseminating information and instruction about dental health. Prior to the institution of the NHS, 5,000 Approved Societies provided dental benefits for about Fourteen Million members, that is three-quarters of the insured population, but because of the cost only a small proportion of these sought treatment until 1948. Then came the deluge; people who had remained edentulous and without dentures because of the cost, and others who for the same reason had had to tolerate broken and ill-fitting vulcanite dentures, crowded dentists' waiting rooms.

By this time all the dental schools had become university departments funded by the University Grants Commission, which demanded full-time teachers, and therefore specialisation. During the war periodontology had received a boost when in 1943 hygienists were trained and used in the Women's Auxiliary Air Force (WAAF), and granted certification by the Ministry of Health in 1949, a development in which G. H. Leatherman DMD LDSRCS, played a very important part. Although South African, Leatherman was trained at Harvard Dental School, and on qualification in 1924 he came to London to obtain the LDS. At his viva his examiner, Kelsey Fry, asked him what he considered to be the most important aspect of dental practice he had brought back from his training in the USA. Without hesitation Leatherman replied , "The practice of oral hygiene." Some years later Kelsey Fry toured the USA and was convinced that Leatherman was right. The association between these two men continued when in 1942 Kelsey Fry was a consultant to the RAF Dental Branch in which Leatherman served. With the then Director of the Branch, Air Vice-Marshal Gordon Ballantyne, Kelsey Fry planned to train dental hygienists at the Medical Training Establishment in Sidmouth, and Leatherman and James Smith were put in charge of a sixteen week training course.

Subsequently Leatherman went on to greater prominence, becoming Secretary-General of the FDI after Fish's triumphant Congress of 1952, and then being elected to the Board of the Faculty of Dental Surgery at the Royal College of Surgeons.

In 1948 a few interested men, including Leatherman, Cross, Wade, the Canadian, Sam Cripps, and Cyril de Vere Green, Consultant Dental Surgeon at the University College Hospital Dental School, met to discuss the foundation of a society. Leatherman wrote to the Deans of all the dental schools to send a representative to a meeting to discuss undergraduate education in oral hygiene, preventive dentistry, and periodontal practice. Nine schools responded, and at last conditions were right for the foundation of a specialist society, the British Society of Periodontology.

At that time ARPA was the active European periodontal society with its own journal, Paradentologie, and George Cross felt that Britain should join this international organisation. To sound out the view of the profession he wrote a letter to the BDJ dated January 7th. 1949, proposing an English section of ARPA. As he reported in the BSP booklet, The First Fifty Years, the letter elicited a good response, including a telephone call from Gerald Leatherman, who invited Cross to have lunch with Dr. Fish and himself. Through the FDI, Fish and Leatherman had become close friends and professional allies, and as Secretary-General of the FDI, Leatherman was in a strong position to understand the political position. In the German section of ARPA there were men who had supported Hitler, and so soon after the war still maintained National Socialist leanings. Leatherman and Fish felt that it was too soon to have relations with such people, and that a British society was needed.

Despite the fact that there were so few full-time teachers of the subject (perhaps only two, Cross and Wade) and no university Chairs, there were a large number of men, senior in the profession throughout the country, who believed that periodontology was an important field, and one which would alter the practice of dentistry. Cyril de Vere Green was appointed as chairman of an ad hoc committee to decide on the constitution and organisation of the proposed society. The Constitution stated that the aim of the Society was 'to promote and advance all aspects of periodontology'.

Fish's book, Parodontal Disease, had appeared in 1944, and had a great impact on teaching in British dental schools. As a student Wade was strongly influenced by Fish's methods and persuaded his teachers at Leeds Dental School to introduce Fish's treatment techniques into the curriculum and to purchase Fish's gingivectomy knives.

Fish was then Chairman of the Dental Board, and therefore an 'additional member' of the GMC, and as such the most influential representative of the profession. He was unanimously elected the first President of the new society with George Cross as the first Honorary Secretary. The first treasurer was Fred Hopper, a protegee of Bradlaw's at Newcastle, and who was to become the Dean of Leeds Dental School. According to Wade, as treasurer, Hopper had to open a bank account for the society. The word periodontology was not known to the bank manager, but after some dictionary research he decided that the word was derived from 'period' and 'ontology', and therefore the society was something to do with planning to be the first men on the moon!

After Fish's period as President, in which the society grew rapidly from its original thirty nine members and associate members, and incorporated 'corresponding' members, that is from other European countries and the colonies, Cyril de Vere Green became President, and subsequently Fish played little part in the society's development. He was always there for advice and as an inspiration, but by 1951 he was very involved in two major activities. At the Dental Board he was preparing for the establishment of a General Dental Council, which would further the autonomy of the profession, and at the FDI he was planning the XIth. Dental Congress of 1952, of which he was to be President Also by 1950 his divorce from Hilda Gertrude had come through, and he was able to marry the widow, Hazel Myfanwy Bruce Hodge. By coincidence Gerald Leatherman was married at the same time.

On 30th. July 1947 the Faculty of Dental Surgery had been

brought into being with Bradlaw as its first Dean and Professor Wilkinson as Vice-Dean In the following year Professor Wilkinson replaced Bradlaw with Kelsey Fry as Vice-Dean, and in turn Fish, who had been elected to the Board in 1950, became Vice-Dean and then Dean in 1956. That was the year in which Fish's great aspiration and that of the whole dental profession was realised with the establishment, at long last, of the General Dental Council. Fish was now sixty-two and had been in the driving seat for many years. His hands were too full to take in active part in the affairs of the BSP, but in 1957 the BSP set up an essay prize out of its funds to encourage undergraduates in periodontology, This came to be replaced by the Sir Wilfred Fish Research Prize awarded annually on the merit of original research on a periodontal subject by a young investigator. Initially the prize was worth £20, awarded in 1972 to Ian C. MacKenzie for his research under the guidance of one of Fish's students, Professor A.E.W. (Loma) Miles at the Department of Oral Pathology, the London Hospital Dental School on 'The Effect of Friction on the Keratinising Epithelia of the Oral Mucosa and Skin of Rodents'. Immediately on completing this research MacKenzie obtained a post at the University of Iowa, adding to the brain drain to the USA.

The BSP always gave education the highest priority, and Messrs. Gibbs provided much financial support for educational matters, especially in relation to the Gibbs Travelling Scholarships awarded to postgraduates and teachers. In this sponsorship H. Colin Davis, Director of Gibbs Oral Hygiene Service, played an important role, and in retirement, Fish in an interview with Davis, gave a fascinating account of his work and thinking.

The BSP prospered, and to celebrate the 25th. anniversary of the Society Fish was invited to be President for the second time, the first occasion on which a president was asked to serve a second term, and in tribute to Fish's early research the main theme of this Silver Jubilee meeting was 'The Clinical Application of Microscopic Studies in Periodontology' The meeting was held at the Royal College of Surgeons in the first week of September, 1974, but on the 20th. July, Fish who had been ill for some time with prostate cancer, died at his home in Storrington, West Sussex.

Fish had inspired the programme for the meeting, to which several eminent overseas speakers were invited. The meeting, attended by over 300 members and guests, was a considerable success, and like the very existence of the Society, a tribute to Fish's role in developing Periodontology as a recognised speciality within dentistry.

Chapter 16

THE DEPARTMENT OF DENTAL SCIENCE

The intention of the Board of the Faculty of Dental Surgery was to set up a research department which would work closely with the Basic Science department of the College, its work directed "towards the application of basic scientific knowledge to dental problems and towards bringing modern methods of investigation to bear on those basic science problems which are peculiar to dentistry itself."

This Department of Dental Science was to be one of eight scientific departments housed in the post-war College, and staffed by full-time research workers. The College agreed to make space available for the new laboratories on the side of the premises overlooking Portugal Street, and adjacent to the Odontological Museum. But the College could not undertake to finance the new department, and the Faculty of Dental Surgery accepted this responsibility.

Fish had been involved in fund raising for research during his years at the Hampton Hale Laboratory and at St. Mary's Meyerstein Laboratory, and he was instrumental in setting up a powerful appeals committee under the Chairmanship of Mr. (later Sir) Walker Shepherd to provide funds for the new department. The committee was set up on January 3rd. 1955, at a luncheon presided over by the College President, Sir Harry Platt. The Committee consisted of members of the Board of the Faculty and city financiers recruited from the ranks of their patients. Gerald Leatherman, then Chairman of the Faculty's Finance Committee, was a driving force. He and Fish, now close friends, made a formidable duo in their ambition for the enterprise, and the Committee was to become a model for a College Appeals Committee, which subsequently collected almost two million pounds for the College. An elegant appeals brochure was sent out to industry, commerce and finance asking for funds to equip and maintain the new Department of Dental Science at the Royal

College of Surgeons. After some years the Dental Faculty's Appeal Committee was merged with that of the College, which then took over the responsibility for financing the Department. Although this provided continuing support for the Department, it did mean loss of independence. In the eleventh 'Sir Wilfred Fish Memorial Lecture' given by Cohen on September 25, 1990, he quoted Leatherman's opinion that, "It is my experience that money creates independence and to a degree every successful research department should have some independence." Leatherman might well have predicted the sad consequences of that loss of independence.

During Wilkinson's term as Dean, Lord Nuffield in 1956 endowed a Nuffield Chair of Dental Research in the Faculty with a trust fund of £100,000. And in that year, when the GDC finally came into being under his Presidency, Fish took over as the Dean of the Faculty. He had in his hands the reins to drive dental research, and by this time, thanks to the Nuffield Foundation's scholarships and fellowships, research was becoming an integral element of the activity of dental schools.

Funding was always a problem, as illustrated by a statement issued by the Finance Committee of the College, which endorsed the desirability of wives accompanying overseas examiners, because of the 'ambassadorial nature' of such visits, but turned down applications to cover wives' expenses.

Further good news came when the Leverhulme Trust decided to provide £6,000 for seven years to fund a research team, and Dr. Bertram Cohen, who had been teaching periodontology and oral pathology in Johannesburg, was appointed Leverhulme Research Fellow in Oral Pathology with effect from November 1956. The appeal for funding had produced promises of about £100,000 over the next seven years. Decisions had to be made about the nature and scope of the research.

By the time of his appointment Cohen's knowledge and experience extended beyond the limits of oral pathology that he had been teaching in South Africa. In 1955 he had been awarded a Cecil John Adams Scholarship to the Postgraduate Medical School at the Hammersmith Hospital where he had worked in the

Pathology department. In his time there he had performed a substantial number of post-mortem examinations, and news of this uniquely experienced dentist came through to Fish from Leatherman. The latter was a member of the American Dental Society of London, the secretary of which was the highly respected prosthodontist, Hamish Thomson, who, by chance, had been a fellow postgraduate of Cohen's at Northwestern Dental School in Chicago. Knowing that Fish needed an oral pathologist Leatherman arranged for a meeting with Cohen, who was encouraged by Fish to apply for the post.

It was the start of a close personal and working relationship, which was to become the secure backbone of the Department of Dental Science, Cohen succeeding Fish as Director. Cohen's general experience was apparent when biopsy material from an apical radiolucency in an elderly lady came into the laboratory. An abundance of giant cells led Cohen to suspect the presence of a parathyroid tumour. This was corroborated by a high blood calcium level and at the subsequent operation performed by Arthur Dickson Wright, who in 1960 became Vice-President of the Royal College of Surgeons, Cohen's suspicions were proved to have been well founded.

Once Fish and Cohen had assumed their appointments, a separate bank account for the department had been opened, and in March 1957 temporary accommodation in the basement of the College, the old dining room, washing-up room and housekeeper's store room, was allocated to the department. One office and a borrowed laboratory was the start, but by April it had expanded to three laboratories. The department paid the College £1,000 annually to cover overheads, and grants came to the department from a variety of sources including the British Empire Cancer Campaign which donated for cancer research £900 as a recurrent annual grant plus a £635 non-recurrent grant. A gift of £2,500 per year for three years was given to provide for a biochemist and technical assistant. In his writing Fish had emphasised the importance of collagen, and was keen to find someone with expertise in this field. His colleague at St. Mary's, Professor Neuberger, a renowned protein scientist, recommended as someone who would fit Fish's need, the young biochemist, Dr. John Eastoe, and in November 1957 Eastoe was appointed, initially for three years at an annual salary of £1,500. He found that when he joined the department the building was in such a state of chaos that the only way to get from one part of it to another was to go through the basement; nevertheless the department was now a going concern.

By this time radio-isotopes had an established place in medicine; carbon-14 was being used to study metabolic processes, thyroid activity could be estimated using iodine-131, and other isotopes were employed in the location of tumours. Fish was very keen to exploit their use in dental research, and one of Cohen's first duties was to go on a radio-isotope course at Harwell. Cohen was appointed Radiation Protection Officer to the College, and he was now well qualified to report on the limitations of the safety precautions in the various departments, including his own.

By April 1959, as Fish was approaching retirement, the new laboratory block on the south side of the College had been completed, and into that excellent accommodation the Department moved with six scientific staff and five auxiliary workers. It was officially opened on the 22nd. May, and the expenses involved in opening the department came to £275 paid out of the department account.

Financial contributions were always welcome, and Fish was approached by an elderly dentist, Frederick Moser, who sought a means of expressing his gratitude to dentistry for the career he had enjoyed over a period of over fifty years. Fish suggested that he should endow a fellowship for a young man wishing to embark on dental research at the Royal College of Surgeons. Moser accepted this suggestion with alacrity, but rather than have his own name attached to the benefaction, he wished to commemorate the kindness that he had received as a poor student from the chairman of the Board of Governors of the Royal Dental Hospital. Thus was created the Quintin Hogg Fellowship to which was added, after Moser's death, the Florence Mills Fellowship in memory of his wife. In October of that year

W.H. Bowen M.Sc., who was to play a major role in caries research, was appointed the Quintin Hogg Fellow for one year, initially at a stipend of £1,200, and Norman Thomas was appointed as Research Assistant.

Fish's ideas about the work of the new department are set out in his paper, 'An Enterprise in Dental Research', which appeared in the *Annals of the Royal College of Surgeons* in May 1958, and therefore, as was characteristic of Fish, was probably written well before the opening of the department. In this he spelt out the attributes he would hope to find in a research worker. Obviously the person (and in this article that person is always male) should have a good grounding in the basic sciences, a logical mind capable of formulating a problem clearly and concisely, and possess the ability to recognise what is important and what is irrelevant. He waxed eloquent on the importance of curiosity and enthusiasm, and what was said of his old teacher of physics, Rutherford, "a kind of instinctive insight".

Fish emphasised the role of prevention, which required understanding of the pathogenesis of the dental diseases, especially what he called the 'periodontal syndrome'. By this statement he recognised the innate variation in individuals in their susceptibility to periodontal disease. Inevitably he wrote about the interdental ulcer. When discussing the cause of caries, he speculated about whether the presence of keratin in stagnation areas, tooth fissures and below the contact point, possibly provided a foothold for acidogenic bacteria.

Many of the themes in this paper were extended in a further paper, 'Research in Clinical Science', which appeared two years later in the *International Dental Journal*. In addition to curiosity and enthusiasm, other qualities were needed in a research worker; the capacity for hard work, tenacity of purpose, a clear and logical brain "which are not characteristics always found in the ardent lover - except perhaps tenacity of purpose", a faculty for concentration on abstract problems and scientific imagination. Of all these curiosity comes first. Fish could well have been describing himself.

In these wide ranging articles, as was always his habit (no

doubt derived from his education at Kingswood School), his quotations range from Vesalius and Galen, through the Curies to the people of his own time, his colleagues at St. Mary's, Almroth Wright and Alexander Fleming, and the role chance played in their discoveries. He quoted Pasteur's famous dictum that "chance only favours the prepared mind." Almroth Wright had seen that a drop of nasal secretion falling on to a bacterial culture in a Petri dish had inhibited bacterial growth, an event replicated when the spore of a mould blew into Fleming's laboratory. Fish's work never seems to have been favoured by such chance events. No such romantic element had entered his years of hard work, which were characterised by minute observation, detailed analysis, logic and burning the midnight oil.

'Research in Clinical Science' is one of the most eloquent of all Fish's papers and was received with great acclaim. As always he made vivid use of analogy, one well remarked example of which was his likening of the qualities of a good research worker to those of a lover. Fish received many letters of congratulations and praise, and Loma Miles was prompted to write, "I thought particularly delightful your analysis of courtship into curiosity and enthusiasm, and your comparison of this happy state with that of the dedicated research worker. Following this line of thought there might be some advantage in enforcing celibacy upon our academic staff in the hope that enthusiasm for one pursuit might be sublimated into the other!"

Fish's attention to detail applied to the provisions for his new research department, and he knew that in his absence he could rely on Cohen to defend the needs of the laboratories and the workers. The building works had included reconstruction of the bomb-damaged old building and additional new building. Construction of the latter, called Phase III A and B, space had to be shared between the various research laboratories plus a television studio and rooms for the secretarial staff which was shared between the departments.

Each department had worked out its own needs for space, and the Building Committee allocated space in Phase IIIB according to the following priority:

The joint secretariat needed 2,000 sq.ft., biochemistry 3,000 sq.ft., pharmacology 3,500 sq.ft., the isotope laboratory, 500 sq.ft., plus space for the television studio.

Fish was away at the time (August 1957), and Cohen pointed out that this added up to a total of 9,000 sq.ft, while the total area of IIIB was only 4,500 sq.ft.

All departments agreed that their requirements needed to be radically pruned, and Cohen was concerned to protect the space allocated to the dental department, as were the heads of all the other research departments. A great deal of horse-trading was needed. Thus, the anatomist, Professor Causey, agreed to give up the fourth floor of the old building in exchange for 1,500 sq.ft. in IIIB, which would join up with his allocated space in the previously completed Phase IIIA.

Cohen reported to Fish that "avaricious glances" were directed towards to the space allocated for dental research, and it was suggested that the dental department's biochemist be housed in the biochemistry laboratory. Although Cohen was resigned to losing some space, he was loathe to give up the bacteriological laboratory because this was one of the few rooms with an outside window providing a pleasant view onto Portugal Street.

The Odontological Museum, essentially Colyer's legacy where Miles was then the Honorary Curator, enjoyed both considerable space and sentimental attachment, and it was generally agreed that the Museum could not be moved. No one wanted to sacrifice laboratory space for the secretariat, and eventually it was agreed that the joint secretarial area be reduced to 1,200 sq.ft.

Fish had earlier suggested that an additional floor be added to IIIB, and this idea was resurrected, the architects being told to go away and do their arithmetic again. In the meantime the basement laboratory was brought into action. Even then this was not achieved without difficulty, and Cohen had to insist that temporary power points be installed to allow incubators to be used. The pace was slow and Cohen was worried that the two young girls employed as laboratory assistants (Fish always called them 'chits') had no work to do.

Away from the department and before departing for a holiday in Italy, Fish was busy designing a table top for the department office, in deal with oak facing. As Cohen describes him, Fish was never one to be constrained by the customary, and the desk was to be S-shaped so that Cohen and Fish could sit side-by-side, but facing one another with their microscopes; the design of the table evidence of Fish's regard for his successor.

Despite all these problems the research staff got off to a reasonable start, and the early publications from the department indicated the broad scope of its research, Cohen reporting on pathology of the salivary glands and secondary tumours of the mandible, and Eastoe on biochemical features of human oral epithelium.

The interdental col became a pre-occupation for both Fish and Cohen, and models were built to demonstrate the failure of the embryonic reduced enamel epithelium to be adequately replaced by keratinised oral epithelium, thus producing a microscopic epithelial ulcer, the initial site of periodontal disease. Fish was given a wonderful opportunity to expound the col theory when in 1959 he was interviewed on television by the celebrity Lady Barnett on the topic, 'The fight against dental disease'. He had taken to the studio models showing the interdental gingiva with the col well defined between the peaks of the gingival margin. On being asked about the early symptoms of gingival disease he described bleeding from the interdental ulcer, which he had successfully treated over a period of 25-30 years by brushing both teeth and gums with a soft toothbrush, thus improving the blood supply to the gums. This, he stressed, was especially important in children. The toothbrush should not only clean the area between the teeth, but should promote growth of the gum between the teeth so that the interdental ulcer healed. He recommended that 20-39 gentle strokes of the brush were needed on either side of the teeth, this brushing carried out twice a day. He did not recommend the use of interdental sticks to produce keratinisation, as he would have done twenty years earlier.

Articles were written and lectures given by Fish and Cohen on the col theory and the interdental ulcer, but the theory was controversial and met with a great deal of opposition. The matter arose when Dr. Henry Goldman, at that time the doyen of American periodontists, visited London. At a meeting at the Eastman Dental Hospital, Bowen heard Goldman and Fish in a heated discussion. Goldman had asked Fish how he could explain the involvement of embryonic tissues where a patient was found to have no periodontal disease at one examination but six months later on subsequent examination, was found to have bone loss. This, it seems, provoked Fish to reply that the patient had not been examined thoroughly in the first place, an answer that could only have antagonised Goldman. The col theory received little support in American texts.

In going through the literature, Cohen found that there seemed to be an antagonistic relationship between calcium and zinc in the production of keratin. This set him wondering if calcium loaded calculus in the interdental area might retard epithelial maturity by inhibiting keratinisation of the col epithelium, and that this might be rectified by the introduction of zinc into the diet of laboratory rats. Subsequently a variety of experiments to study the behaviour of interdental epithelium were carried out on monkeys. Laboratory animals were given code names, such as Bing and Ding, the vowel 'I' indicating that the animal was a monkey, and the letters 'NG' denoted that it had had a gingivectomy. This caused much hilarity at meetings of the International Association of Dental Research where the findings were reported.

Cohen's seniority in the College was established when he was given authority by the College to accept the invitation of the South East Metropolitan Regional Hospital Board to take up the appointment of Honorary Consultant Surgeon in Dentistry at the Queen Victoria Hospital in East Grinstead. This position gave Cohen the opportunity to set up a biopsy service for diagnosing specimens of oral pathology. With the assistance of Colin Smith and later of Martin Edwards, this service flourished and rendered valuable diagnosis to patients in the hospitals making use of this biopsy service. Both Smith and Edwards, assiduous workers, completed doctoral theses based on research into the diagnosis of malignant disease in the mouth. This biopsy service was to bear unexpected fruit when Cohen retired.

Fish's protegees and friends were also given recognition when Beric Southwell, one of Fish's partners in practice in Sevenoaks was elected to the Board of the Faculty of Dental Surgery, and Gerald Leatherman was appointed Vice-Dean. In the same year Dr. RichardtenCate, who was to go on to become Vice-Chancellor of the University of Toronto, was appointed to the Leverhulme Fellowship in Dental Research to the Department for three years at a salary of £1,650 rising to £1,850.

By 1961, Fish's first year in retirement, much to Cohen's and Fish's delight, five staff members of the department gave papers at the annual meeting of the International Association for Dental Research (IADR). These included ten Cate, Bowen and Norman Thomas, all of whom proceeded to considerable professional success, and Ted Brain, who had started as a research technician in the department and went on to obtain his M.Sc.

In 1959, on relinquishing the post of Dean of the Faculty of Dental Surgery, Fish resigned from his seat as co-opted member of the College Council, his place being taken by Professor Martin Rushton of Guy's. But despite his approaching retirement, Fish kept up with his many other commitments. As the President of the GDC, he proposed the toast to the School and Hospital at the Centenary Dinner of the Royal Dental Hospital, which was attended by H.M.Queen Elizabeth, the Queen Mother, at which he recalled, perhaps tongue in cheek, his many happy days spent as a member of staff. In that year he became the President of the IADR, had enjoyed (as described) the television interview with the TV personality of those days, Lady Barnett, and was appointed Honorary Consultant to the Army. But the most important event of the year was the Centenary celebrations of the first dental diploma.

In his address, Fish said, "It was a hundred years since Queen Victoria granted the Council of the Royal College of Surgeons, which was already an examining body in general surgery, a Royal Charter permitting them to examine persons desirous of being so examined and to issue certificates of fitness to practise dentistry." And to commemorate the occasion Fish presented the Faculty with a fine silver cup dated 1751. Quintin Hogg's grandson, Lord Hailsham, then Minister of Health, proposed the toast to the Faculty, and as Fish commented, "He was unable to forgo a passing reference to the merits of conservative dentistry, but preserved an appearance of political impartiality in promising more liberal support for more radical research." Fish was furious that Hailsham had not acknowledged the strides that had been made in dental research, and in his notes on the event he wrote, "Hailsham had been badly briefed and groaned about dentistry's lack of research - oblivious of the new department for which we had collected a quarter of a million pounds without MRC help - when he sat down I told him that his remarks had cost him £1,000 a year, and next day wrote for a grant for a new research assistant wanted- and got it!"

In that year Fish gave one of his most frequently quoted lectures, "A Profession in the Making." and in describing the history of the profession this lecture followed the theme of his talk, 'The Englishman's Teeth' , given almost twenty years earlier. Fish had ended this lecture by promoting the idea of a hospital for clinical research and post-graduate teaching. That aspiration was being fulfilled in the developing activity of the dental schools as university departments. The Department of Dental Science represented dentistry's move into the basic biological sciences, and despite financial constraints, in Fish's four years at the helm it had made a promising start. As he wrote in 1960 in a letter to The Times on the subject of research, "find first of all the men, then the money."

Fish recognised the talent needed to make an effective research team, and when surrounded by his staff in a department which represented the fruits of his dream and his labours, he must have known a sense of considerable satisfaction. Those who worked with him at the Department of Dental Science, such as Bert Cohen and John Eastoe, found a relaxed and happy man. Eastoe describes an occasion at coffee time when with his staff around him, Fish became very excited and in great good humour spun round on his chair so that the spindle came loose, and Eastoe had to catch the flying Fish! He was certainly a man content with himself.

Fish was in regular touch with the Nuffield organisations, and a letter of September 1959 from G. McLachlan, secretary of The Nuffield Provincial Hospital Trust says." ..even an informal conversation over dinner can go a long way towards constructive proposals.... and the time is ripe for a review of all the problems facing dentistry."

As the department grew it took in research workers who had obtained Nuffield Fellowships, and proved to be the nursery of many prominent in dental teaching, research and administration.

In November 1960 Fish retired as Honorary Director of the Department, Cohen taking his place. Fish had stated quite clearly that he would not follow the examples of Kelsey Fry and Wilkinson, who it seems could not keep away from Lincoln's Inn Fields, and except for attending Faculty dinners his appearances at the College were rare. He and Cohen kept in close touch throughout Fish's retirement, Cohen providing information about research in progress at the Department and what was reported at meetings of the IADR. Fish felt assured that the department was in good hands, and that the quality of the research, with Eastoe and Bowen now in harness under Cohen's direction, would fulfil his expectations. He was now sixty-six and still vigorously involved in his responsibilities as President of the GDC, as well as in other matters.

Dickson Wright met Fish six months after he retired, and remarked to Cohen that Fish looked years younger and sun-tanned, "I thought that he would pine away and die when he retired." When Cohen relating this to Fish complimented him on retiring so successfully, the latter replied, "..not really, old boy. When I retired I vowed that within six months, if anyone said , 'teeth', I'd think of a comb. But dammit I still think of the Mouth."

Soon after Fish's retirement Cohen was able to appoint two new junior Fellows, George Camilleri, a brilliant graduate from Malta who was working at the Glasgow Dental School, and Colin Smith a recent graduate from the Royal Dental Hospital. These two new additions forged an excellent partnership, each engaged on research directed towards the early detection of oral cancer.

Each enjoyed considerable success during their fellowships, Smith obtaining a Ph.D, and brought distinction to the Department in their subsequent careers, each becoming Dean of a dental school, Camilleri in Malta and Smith in Sheffield. It was a matter of great satisfaction to Fish that the Department began to attract more and more visiting research fellows from all over the world, including New Zealand, Australia, Canada, South Africa, Switzerland, Scandinavia, Israel and Finland.

Negotiations with the Nuffield Foundation continued and these culminated in the Nuffield Foundation Conference on Assistance to Academic Dentistry held on 22-24 February 1963 at Ashridge College in Hertfordshire.

The conference was attended by 73 people, a galaxy of dental stars, many former Nuffield Fellows and Scholars, and now holding positions of influence in dental teaching and research. It was felt that after nearly twenty years of Nuffield Foundation support an opportunity to meet would be the best way of guiding the Foundation in its future assistance to academic dentistry. Fish, as President of the GDC, and Bradlaw as Dean of the Institute of Dental Surgery at the Eastman Dental Hospital, attended. In summing up, Cohen spoke of the need to give people incentives to do research, and to provide them with good prospects and good research facilities, including laboratory animals, especially monkeys. Thus he anticipated the development of the primate colony at Downe Research Centre, which Fish and Cohen were keen to establish.

In expressing his thanks to the meeting, Fish said, "... as the senior member, I must have had longer experience of dentistry than anyone else in this room ," and he continued to speak of the need for high quality dental teachers, to which end headmasters and science sixth formers must be persuaded that there is a future in dentistry for those young people at the top of the science sixth and not at the bottom. It had become one of his favourite themes.

Over the next twenty years the research at the Department progressed under Cohen's direction, with Bowen looking at the possibility of producing a vaccine against Streptococcus Mutans, and Eastoe continuing his work on the collagen matrix of enamel.

But other new avenues were also explored. Richard tenCate introduced histochemical techniques into the Department and used this tool to explore the distribution of various enzymes in the oral tissues, and this work was taken up and expanded by A. H. Melcher, a South African graduate, whose chief interest was in the connective tissues of the gingiva and periodontium. He was largely responsible for introducing electron microscope techniques to the Department, and initiated a useful collaboration with workers in the Electron Microscopy Unit of the Imperial Cancer Research laboratories which adjoined the College. At the conclusion of his tenure of a Leverhulme Fellowship he, like tenCate, emigrated to Canada where he became Director of the Canadian Medical Council Periodontal Research Unit.

As the research programme expanded accommodation at Lincoln's Inn Fields became more and more cramped, but as a consequence of the Ashridge Conference the Nuffield Foundation came to the rescue with a grant to erect new laboratories if a suitable site could be found. The election to the Presidency of the College of Sir Arthur (later Lord) Porritt, an old friend of Sir Wilfred's from his days at St. Mary's Hospital, facilitated the provision of a plot of land at Downe in Kent, adjoining the home of Charles Darwin. In 1966 the new laboratories and animal house were officially opened by Fish and glowing tributes were paid to his fundamental contribution to the enterprise by Lord Brock who had succeeded Porritt as President, and by Sir Terence Ward, then Dean of the Faculty of Dental Surgery. Fish later described this as one of the happiest days in his professional life.

The creation of the research unit at Downe provided new impetus to the Department. A veterinary scientist, Dr. Charles Coid, joined the staff and was largely responsible for designing a primate colony. While still at Lincoln's Inn Fields, Cohen and Bowen had run a pilot study on a small group of macaque monkeys and had shown that dental caries exactly similar to that seen in humans could be produced in these animals when they were maintained on a diet high in fermentable carbohydrate. Under Coid's guidance a highly successful system of caging and animal husbandry soon resulted in a flourishing breeding and experimental macaque colony that aroused interest from various scientific disciplines in many parts of the world. Among those attracted to the opportunities provided was David Poswillo, a new Zealand oral surgeon whose work on cleft palate in rats had been recognised as outstanding. Awarded a Nuffield Fellowship in order to spend a year in the U.K., Poswillo soon established himself and at the termination of his fellowship the College offered him a permanent position as Professor of Teratology. To support his research the well known charity, Action for the Crippled Child, provided additional funding to enlarge the Dental Research Unit in order to add research laboratories and a marmoset breeding colony along similar lines to the macaque programme. The shorter period of gestation of these small South American primates made them more suitable for teratological research. In subsequent years there followed significant research on congenital anomalies and facial deformities, including a conclusive demonstration of the teratogenic mechanism of thalidomide.

Concurrently activity in the macaque colony was largely devoted to caries research, work by Bowen on a vaccine having got off to a highly promising start. However this was not matched by subsequent progress, until the advent of Dr. Geoffrey Colman, a dental graduate who had left clinical practice to study microbiology. He replaced Bowen, who had been the first to hold the position, as Wilfred Fish Research Fellow. This title had been approved by the Council of the College to commemorate the founding father of the Department. Colman's arrival brought new impetus to this project and with the arrival of Roy Russell, a biochemist, a period of scientific productivity ensued. For a time it appeared that the holy grail of caries prevention by vaccination was within reaching distance, but the risks of complications arising from vaccine therapy were difficult to justify for the prevention of non-lethal disease. Moreover there were limits to the generous support from outside bodies and this imposed restrictions on the recruitment of personnel. Colman was appointed to a high position in the Public Health Laboratory

Service at Colindale, and soon after Russell succeeded Eastoe as Professor of Oral Biology at the University of Newcastle, so that by the time of Cohen's retirement in 1983 the Department was understaffed and College finances too depleted to do much about it. Despite continuing and generous support from the Nuffield Foundation, the Chocolate and Confectionery Alliance, and the Sugar Association, for matters of finance and personnel the Department was no longer an independent entity within the College. Its finances were in the control of the College, and as Gerald Leatherman had opined many years earlier, loss of financial independence puts research at risk A further signal of the diminished role of the Department was the appointment of Professor Newell Johnson to succeed Cohen as Nuffield Professor. Johnson was already a very busy man, holding the Chair of Oral Pathology at the London Hospital Dental School, as well as being appointed to head an MRC unit to pursue research into periodontal disease.

At about this time Imperial College incorporated St. Mary's Hospital Medical School and Professor Sir Stanley Peart FRS, formerly Professor of Medicine at the school and from 1988 - 92 Master of the Hunterian Institute, the teaching arm of the Royal College of Surgeons, was delegated to rationalise various research programmes at the College. His decision was to dismantle the Department of Dental Science. The Department may have continued to possess a constitutional existence but after 1993 it no longer had a home in Lincoln's Inn Fields where its history belongs, with Fish as its inspiration and Cohen its Director for over twenty years.

From then, due to further hospital reorganisation, Newell Johnson has sat behind Fish's old desk, but not at the Royal College of Surgeons nor at the London Hospital, but at King's College Hospital Dental School where Johnson continues research on oral cancer. The desk has made a journey that no one could have predicted, and fortunately, one that Fish was not to witness.

The year before he retired Cohen was awarded a CBE in the New Year's Honours List and on retirement a new and welcome challenge presented itself. He was invited by the Imperial Cancer Research Fund to recruit retired pathologists to a histopathology unit to deal with enquiries about biopsy examination and diagnosis. This group came to be known as the Wise Men. If Fish had been alive he would have been delighted that such an unexpected shoot had stemmed from the biopsy service provided by the Department, but he would have derived most satisfaction from the knowledge that his inspiration had become, under Cohen's muscular direction, a recruiting and training ground for some of the most distinguished people in dentistry in many countries throughout the world. Fish had not been either a university professor nor the Dean of a dental school, but through the Department he was the patriarch and major influence to many who came after him.

Chapter 17

IN RETIREMENT

Perhaps retirement is the wrong word to describe Fish's staged withdrawal from his official positions and professional activity. The hats he wore were shed one by one; first the Honorary Directorship of the Department of Dental Science which was taken over by Professor Cohen, then practice in Cavendish Square, already run by Stewart Ross and colleagues, and finally, twenty years after he had been appointed Chairman of the Dental Board, retirement from the Presidency of the General Dental Council to be succeeded on the 1st March 1965 by Professor Sir Robert Vivian Bradlaw. Fish had the satisfaction of knowing that he had left his professional heritage in safe hands.

He had given much thought to the prospect of retirement, sometimes seen as attractive and at others rather daunting. In some undated notes, possibly written well before retiring, he ruminated on the subject in a way that would have surprised many of his colleagues:

"Tired of the struggle - achieved a degree of fulfilment - so why not retire to seek peace. Tired. Lie back and retire.- peace - you think - you've always thought - don't think - peace. You think how pleasant not to have to think".

"Each day to rest - don't think - you sleep. You wake refreshed - again you think - you always have - it's odd, you can't just not think. You get a small place - less work, less to think about - except the garden - got to have a garden. But that's not work. That's relaxation. Couch grass, ground-elder , dandelion, clover. Just naturalize it - a few flowers , a little lawn and deck chair, peace, think how to kill the weeds - You always have thought. "Don't think how - just do it . What with? Look it up, let the other fellow think. Which way is best? Have to think it out, there you go again. Relax- bliss - weeds - try digging them out. Tired? Yes, very. Must rest and relax and stop thinking. Get a fellow in to do the garden."

So Fish meditated, rather whimsically, on retirement. In truth, he wrote out many such ruminations, because he could as much not write as not think, and in one of these he wrote, "...retirement, like practice, is really a whole-time job, and also, like practice, it takes a whole lot of effort and concentration and thought to prepare for it. A man should start this preparation not later than the day he qualifies. Being somewhat precocious I started before I was seven."

But fifty-nine years later, although ruminating about the benefits of gardening and even playing golf, when Fish retired from the Department of Dental Science, he could not put work, nor thinking about work, behind him.

At the time of Fish's retirement from the Department of Dental Science epidemiological research had shown that a reduction in sweet consumption and improvement in oral hygiene reduced the incidence of dental caries, and that dental health education was an extremely important preventive measure. However inadequacies in the NHS dental service, especially for children, were obvious, and the subject of many parliamentary questions, in particular from three well known members, Barnett (later Lord) Janner, Tom Driberg and Jennie Lee, the wife of Aneurin Bevan. By then the school dental service was only 300 inspectors stronger than it had been a decade earlier. Janner, MP for Leicester, had already raised the fact that the Standing Committee on Dental Health Education was unable to carry on with its work for lack of funds, and in November 1960 he pointed out to the Minister of Education that in Leicester there were 62,000 children with five school dental officers, two of whom were part-time, so that many children had not had a dental inspection for five years. Driberg asked the Minister whether he was aware of the severe incidence of dental caries in school children because of this deficiency. The shortage of dentists was a regular subject of questioning, to which the Minister, then Lord Balniel, pointed to the expansion of several dental schools including King's College Hospital, Bristol, Newcastle, Leeds and Manchester. The McNair Committee recommended that the dental schools increase their output to 800 dentists per year. Fish took a different tack, and as

President of the GDC, wrote to Lord Cohen of Birkenhead, an eminent physician, Professor of Medicine at Liverpool University, and advisor to the Department of Health, expressing the view that " the solution to the caries problem can hardly be tackled by people whose main job is teaching." He also asked Cohen if he could recruit the support of Lord Woolton, who had been Minister of Food in Churchill's wartime Cabinet.

On the 27th July 1960, in the House of Lords, Woolton asked, "..Her Majesty's Government if they will state the figure that is being spent per annum through the Medical Research Council on dental research, and what proportion of that sum, if any, is being spent on the prevention of caries in children, and further, what relation this sum bears to the total government expenditure on medical research, and also, if they can give any estimate of the financial value of the production of sugar confectionery in this country."

The Lord Privy Seal and Minister for Science, the lawyer, Viscount Hailsham, replied that the MRC's current expenditure on dental research amounted to more than £35,000, and he added that the function of the MRC was research not prevention. He went on to say that the value of the home-produced sugar confectionery, including chocolate confectionery, during 1959, was £193 million, and the total consumption came to £259 million. Woolton replied that he wished the Minister's reply had given him greater satisfaction, "of course £35,000 on the subject of dental caries in this country is - I was going to say insignificant; but surely it is ludicrous.... I would ask the noble Viscount... whether he will take any steps to contact the makers of sugar confectionery to see whether by an increase in chemical research, they cannot produce a confectionery which does not cause dental caries. Out of a turnover which the noble Viscount says is £259 million, there must be a great deal of extra profit which they might use to such a noble cause, ..(will he) enquire from them whether they would be prepared to undertake such research."

Hailsham replied that it was not lack of funds but lack of interest and enthusiasm on the part of both dental and scientific graduates. He also pointed out that £750,000 a year was spent on dental work at universities, but he did not specify how much of that went on research.

Another of Their Lordships, Lord Taylor, pointed out that tobacco manufacturers donate to the MRC for research into lung cancer, perhaps the sweet manufacturers could do the same. He also asked whether there was a sufficiency of a career structure to a high enough level in dental research. To this Hailsham replied that there was a lamentable lack of interest in the subject. In this exchange the Department of Dental Science was never mentioned. Fish was furious, and (as described above) when he met Hailsham he pointed out the omission, and said that Hailsham owed him the price of a research worker. A grant duly arrived.

To some extent Hailsham's opinion that not enough dentists were interested in research was justifiable. Earnings in general practice were much higher than in teaching or research, but behind this was the persistent shortage of dentists. The Daily Mirror of 17th March 1961 reported that Britain urgently needed 4,000 more dentists, that the school dental services were 50% understaffed, and that the dentist-population ratio had dropped from 1:3,000 in 1926 to 1:4,000 in 1961.

Fish continued to take the view that more research rather than more dentists was the long-term solution, and he reiterated that the "solution to the caries problem can hardly be tackled by people whose main job is teaching"; it followed therefore that research might be better carried out when not connected with a university. In October 1960 he wrote to his friend, Dr. Senior at the Ministry of Health, with a proposal that he called his 'swan song'. This was to establish a research team to investigate the aetiology and prevention of caries, to be under the auspices of the MRC, but "not diverting funds from other researchers into caries."

Senior's reply was a model of friendly tact, in which he likened Fish's approach to his projects to Montgomery's fighting tactics, that is concentrated hard on a narrow front, unlike Eisenhower's, which were much more broadly based. Senior knew his friend well for Fish was firing on all barrels. He approached Sir Harold Himsworth, Director of the MRC, and suggested meeting for lunch at the Athenaeum. As was always his practice in making his case, he sent Himsworth a very detailed and lengthy memorandum detailing the history of staffing in dental teaching and research.

In 1940 the Medical Mission and other buildings in Bermondsey, a deprived area of London to the south of Tower Bridge, were destroyed by bombing, and a Public Health Centre was being planned on that site. The Member of Parliament for the constituency was Bob Mellish, who had been Labour Chief Whip and Minister of Housing, and Fish approached him with the idea of incorporating a dental clinic and research laboratory in the new Health Centre. He felt that the facilities at the Royal College of Surgeons did not provide the space for the specialised laboratory he envisaged. In March 1961, Fish was given lunch by Mellish at the House of Commons, and they looked over the plans of the Centre, which was spacious enough to give grounds for optimism. In a further paper on what Fish called, the 'Central Institute of Dental Research', he made a comprehensive costing of rent, rates, wages for staff, cost and depreciation of equipment, the Director's expenses, and all other details of expenditure for such an institute which he reckoned would amount to £32,000 a year, and he added that a sum of £40,000 annually should be "held available after the initial period." Also he drew plans of the laboratories and associated facilities in the hypothetical institute, for which he described the Department of Dental Science as "in a sense a prototype."

Fish felt that the scheme should have the Minister of Health's prior approval, and duly wrote to Enoch Powell, whom he had talked to about the need for research when the Minister had opened the New Cross School for Dental Auxiliaries. In order to test the attitude of the MRC to his idea, Fish wrote to Martin Rushton, who was then a member of the MRC's Dental Committee, but Rushton would not commit himself one way or another before the matter came before the committee. However he did suggest that such a research centre should be associated with a university or the Postgraduate Medical Federation, and that it would need a director who "could carry through a new and promising approach to the caries problem." Everyone seemed to be agreed that such a laboratory would be useful, but the general belief was that expansion of the dental schools would provide for such research.

Fish wrote to Mellish, "I am not entirely unhopeful that the Lord will provide."

In May 1961 Fish wrote to Rowntree and Co.Ltd in York about financial support for his scheme, and received a reply from J.E.Chapman, the secretary of The Cocoa, Chocolate and Confectionery Alliance. This was labelled 'confidential', and its contents could have been a model for the tobacco industry in years to come. It read," Clear scientific evidence that sugar and confectionery are a major cause of dental caries in this country has not been found. However the lack of 'unassailable' evidence on the causes of dental caries prevents definite conclusions being reached on the role of confectionery, and leads to the verdict that the case against confectionery is "not proven". The letter added that should a unit be established it should be organised and financed on a national basis, and that their further grant to the MRC would be a help.

In July Lord Woolton agreed to meet Fish at the House of Lords, but whatever might have come from that meeting would have been of little use as in the following month the MRC decided that caries research be related to university dental schools, and in particular the MRC intended to support the work being carried out by Darling at Bristol. Fish's response was predictable; he thought that it was a pity the job could not be done adequately where research workers were handicapped by clinical responsibilities, as they were in Darling's school.

His letter to Bob Mellish clearly expressed his disappointment; "our scheme is a dead horse... it is no good flogging the corpse." An interesting aspect of Fish's endeavours is that he seems not to have discussed this exercise with Cohen. In other matters which maintained his interest Fish kept in regular touch with Cohen, especially about the activity of the department, where Cohen was involved in the setting up a primate colony at the Royal College of Surgeons research establishment at Downe in Kent. Fish continued to ponder on ideas for research, and even in 1967, as shown by a letter written at 3.50 a.m., he wrote to Cohen on how radioactive material might be used in research.

In the same year Fish was approached by a writer, one John Woodforde, who asked for advice because he had been commissioned to write a popular history of false teeth. Woodforde had been told by the famous novelist, Compton Mackenzie, that the war had been won by the partial denture Fish had made for Churchill, because without his four front teeth Churchill's speech was indistinct. Fish replied asking Woodforde not to include the Churchill story because, " any element of truth it may contain has become so distorted as to make it unrecognisable, and ordinary reticence, let alone professional etiquette prevents me from giving any information about Sir Winston's treatment."

Fish's writings and reputation were known world-wide. In August 1969, after a visit to the Soviet Union, Stewart Ross received a letter from Russia in which the writer expressed the view that it was good "to hear from you of Sir Wilfred Fish whom we look upon as the greatest, and describe him in Russian style as the Man with a capital M."

Although Fish continually thought about ideas for research, and even about the genesis of the epithelial attachment, he does not seem to have missed professional activity or committee meetings. Hazel has said that he loved his retirement. These were years of comfortable domesticity in which the family played an important part. His elder sister Nellie was a frequent visitor, but a visit from his beloved South African grand-daughter, James' daughter Patricia, represented a special occasion. Fish and Patricia, had communicated regularly from early in her childhood. Fish's letters, often written in verse, were frequently decorated with little sketches of animals and birds. One verse written with apologies to H.B.(Hilaire Belloc), was sent on receiving a present of two book-marks from Patricia:

Precious Child how could you know,
(for I have never told you so)
that ever since the age of three,
(that's when it first occurred to me)
I found that reading books in pairs
leaves much more time for such affairs
as treating people's teeth and gums
or growing large chrysanthemums?

Like many a more deserving wight
I am endowed with second sight
At least I have two eyes, indeed
With either one can see to read.
So, (while) the one is reading tosh
The other ploughs through something posh.
But now, attend the awful sequel,
My brain bumps are quite unequal.

And as a sequel to the anonymous piece of doggerel;

There was a young fellow said, "Damn!"
I don't like to think that I am
Just a being who moves
In predestinate grooves
Not a bus, not a car but a tram

After much crossing out and little attention to scansion, Fish wrote:

No sir! You're something much
more than a bus or a car or a tram
you have no set up plan like a bus
You just jump on your bike
and go where you like
and for nobody else care a cuss.

Finally in 1962 when she was twelve, Patricia (Trich) and her
mother, now divorced from James, made their first visit to Fish and

Hazel. For Trich, with her 'Gramps' being a Sir and Churchill's dentist, he was also a man with a capital M. By this time the Fish's had moved from Weymouth Street to a house with a garden and the essential greenhouse in Esher. It must have been a wonderful time for Fish, and as Trich writes, " He was full of stories about this and that....there was a stool covered with light blue velvet and silver legs, which Gramps told me, came from Elizabeth II's coronation...(that) stuck to him because he had to sit so long at the ceremony .

"...there was a room at the end of the passage into which no-one was allowed... this was a special room... I later discovered when I was older that it was "the dentist room" where he would go and do dentist things.."

"he had a marvellous sense of humour. My dad (James) told the story of how Gramps would tease Vivienne about dying after eating her pudding - she would then leave her dessert and my dad would happily eat it."

"He always sat at the head of the table, facing the window or the French door so that he could see the birds feeding on the bird feeder that he had rigged up outside. Always made sure the birds had food - apple, crumbs, seed and cheese."

"He would feed the dogs at the table from a fork - which he did to annoy his sister Nellie and much to my amusement."

"I was taught names like 'gazinter' = screwdriver because it goes into the wall, and 'gazunder' - chamber pot because it goes under the bed.."

"He insisted that we hoist the flag every day - very patriotic."

"He also had a bear in the home - a large brown teddy bear called 'Bohuncus'. He allowed me to take it to bed every night and because he was too big to take home to S.A. he gave me a small one for my birthday when we left called 'Josephus' which I still have to this day."

Soon after Trich's visit Fish and Hazel, feeling that Esher was not to their liking because it had become too overcrowded, they moved to Storrington, a quieter place in Sussex woodlands, where they had a bungalow built. As always the garden was one of its most important features, and the Storrington house had a large conservatory where, as Hazel says, "he grew all sorts - experimenting of course! That was his form of gardening. I was the one who designed and tended the garden. That must be my Scotch blood coming out.". The house on Weymouth Street was his only home without a garden, and although Hazel claims that she did all the gardening, the truth is that her husband laboured hard to create his gardens, putting especial effort into landscaping and building the rockeries. Indeed through these labours he became very fit, and those colleagues at the Royal College of Surgeons who had predicted that retirement would kill him, were confounded when faced with a lean and brown man. The Fishs' frequent moves seem to represent an impulse to satisfy this creative bent; once he had completed one garden he felt the need to move to a new challenge. Throughout his life he had enjoyed the physical activity involved in horse riding and rowing, and then deer stalking, and although he was keen on propagating plants the physical activity involved in making a garden seems to have had great appeal; David Poswillo recalls how when he helped Fish to build brick walls in the Storrington garden Fish taught him how to cut paving stones. Cohen and his wife, also Hazel, were themselves keen gardeners and now close friends of Fish and his wife, and the begonias that the Cohens still grow were propagated from Fish's plants. Indeed there was considerable affection between the two men. Loma Miles, Fish's student and then assistant in the Periodontal Department at the RDH, said that Fish was rather aloof even as a young man, and so he seems to have been in some professional situations, but as Trich always recalls that her Gramps was a very generous man, who after James' divorce, was still very supportive of herself and her mother. Cohen and Poswillo and many other have testified that he was capable of great friendship and kindness as well as inspiring great respect and loyalty. After a lecture given by Fish to The American Dental Society of London in 1969, the Honorary Secretary, Hamish Thomson, wrote, " I must write this without the typewriter because there must be feeling in what I say. It is seldom that any of the professions is exalted by a philosophical as well as intellectual appraisal of what it is about."

Fish was given a chance to look back over his life's work when in April 1968, in a series called 'Face-to-Face', the dental newspaper *Dental News* reported an interview by its editor, H.Colin Davis, with Fish at his final home in Storrington, Sussex in August of the year before. The meeting took place on the terrace of the garden that Fish had created by his own exertions on a sloping tract of Sussex woodland. The small retirement home had been built to his own design with a view across acres of silver birch and pine, "with Chanctonbury Ring placed with the eye of an artist in the top left hand corner of the picture. Centre foreground a window box of heathers which he had propagated himself, two glasses dry sherry; and warm spring sunshine provided by the Almighty."

By that time Fish had been in complete retirement for almost three years, time enough to reflect on the importance of the various aspects of a crowded life, and in answer to Davis's question, "What recipe would you give to a member of our profession for a happy retirement?", Fish had his reply ready. He said that he had "tried to compile an inventory of the things I personally thought important. I have put the most important first:

> A job of work - but something that you want to do
> A well grilled steak and teeth to match - the kind that grew
> A glass of wine, perhaps a choice - and maybe two
> A good companion - well tried friend who likes the things that you like too
> And health, and wealth enough to see you through
> A few regrets - the naughty things you did - more tantalizing still the one's you didn't do
> Some credit, somewhere, to reflect upon - and then
> ...a quick release;
> and unperturbed, be gone!"

As with every thing he wrote, including his occasional verse, Fish had prepared a number of earlier drafts of these lines, in particular the last few words. Alternatives had been, ".. and dignified be gone" and "...depart with dignity", but evidently he decided that the subjective requirement of peace of mind was more important than any outward show of dignity. Indeed, as his personal notes show, he had reflected not only on retirement but on the passing of time and death. The certainties of this jocular verse mask the very real uncertainties that are manifest in those other reflections from an earlier date.

Colin Davis' next question, "of the fields in which you worked...which gave you the greatest satisfaction?" has been recorded in an earlier chapter, where Fish replied, "Oh undoubtedly periodontics....(that) was a problem in basic pathology, and in those days one had to start from scratch." In reply to the question, "What do you think are the essential attributes of the successful private practitioner?" Fish enlarged on the importance of a good bedside manner, and the ability to convince the patient that one's interest in them as a person was not simply as a dental problem.

His comment when asked about the NHS dental service demonstrated a clear understanding of the situation which still seems to evade many people. "The State could only hope to provide a basic standard of treatment. It could hardly be expected to provide luxuries... a good amalgam is better than a doubtful inlay."

The interview progressed on predictable lines with Fish recounting student days including his hero, Rutherford, and although Fish was obviously delighted to be interviewed, (later he marked the top of his copy of the newspaper with the words, "exclusive interview - with me!"), perhaps his natural sardonic wit was provoked when asked, " If you had your time over again, would you follow the same diversified pattern?", for he replied, "I am tempted to vary Pontius Pilate's question and ask you, 'What is time?' but I can make my point more simply by the old crack - 'if you had a brother would he like rice pudding?" However he did allow the modest Englishman to appear, adding, " As for my other activities outside practice, apart from research which was my hobby, they were jobs that just happened - one found oneself involved and there it was." This denial of his drive, ambition and energy which had produced so many positive contributions to dentistry, is reminiscent of the sang-froid that he displayed when the troopship taking him to India was sinking beneath his feet. Was this his natural inclination as an English gentleman, or possibly a manifestation of his well developed sense of irony?

As the years went by Fish followed the progress of the research at the Department of Dental Science and the problems involved in building the primate colony at Downe, where Bowen and then Colman worked on a vaccine against caries in primates. In April 1970 Cohen was to write to Fish of Bowen's work, "He ... has made a contribution to caries research which, in my belief, is enough to keep his name in the literature for many decades to come. No one can take away from him the fact that he was the first person, and in fact remains the only person to inoculate a primate against dental caries." This work seemed so promising that the National Institute of Dental Research in Washington made public the claim that, "Victory over caries is in sight."

Since working at St. Mary's Hospital with MacLean on *Streptococcus Viridans,* Fish had believed that an anti-caries vaccine might one day be produced, and he looked forward to the day when Cohen and his department would receive recognition for having solved the twin problems of dentistry, that is the aetiology of periodontal disease, with the col as its centre (Fish was still sceptical of the role of bacterial plaque), and the identification of the micro-organism responsible for caries.

But by this time symptoms of prostate disease had become apparent and cancer was diagnosed, for which oestrogens were prescribed. Fish saw more than one urologist, and in a letter to Cohen he compared one rectal examination with a previous one, as a skilful finger in a rubber glove compared to an iron clad fist.

Surgery was indicated and in May 1970 he was recommended to consult the surgeon, Michael Snell , who, to Fish's delight, was a consultant at St. Mary's Hospital. Fish had been studying the statistics of survival rates and making his own calculations, and after seeing Snell he wrote that " his report gives me a much firmer basis for my own calculations..."

The post-operative period seems to have gone smoothly, and Fish started to put his papers in order. To this end he needed his devoted assistant, Ted Brain, to collect his old slides, and to help sort them out he ordered a viewing box, for which he was happy to send Cohen a cheque.

Despite relative physical inactivity Fish refused to have a television set. The only event he watched was the moon landing, and when Trich came in 1972 she had to "pop in to the dear old lady across the road to watch Top of the Pops." She would accompany him to the local butcher where he bought steaks just for the two of them, and "like a naughty boy" his favourite treacle tart. Meanwhile Hazel continued very busy with her painting and attending art exhibitions. For some years the marriage had not been easy; it seems that Hazel felt that he was not a sympathetic man to live with, and even his granddaughter says that he had to have his own way. "He was a very determined man and a leader and you had to toe the line and fit in with his plans." Unlike Fish's first wife, Hazel was quite capable of being independent.

In some verse Fish reveals a great deal more about his life and his failed first marriage than anything that he recorded in any other form. The following poem is undated but portrays a mood of regret and reconciliation that can only have come late in life.

On Life, Eternity and Reality

The tears that wait on life - are they all shed?
I trust not so. Hearts that never melt all love is dead
The desperate scalding tears
That burnt up hope itself in earlier years
And in whose bitter flow faith too seemed to have drained
away,
Until, of that eternal trinity - faith, hope and Charity (love)
The last alone remained, - those tears have all been shed
and moments of brief happiness regained.
But still hearts melt at mortal woe, and brimming eyes
o'erflow,
What happiness was thrown away!
- yet, had we sought to keep it, who can say

what plans the fates, who tantalise before they slay,
held in suspense, what devastating blow?
No, look not back except in gratitude
For those resplendent days in forest glade that bade us hope.
They lie there still to be relived and they will never fade
The future still may hold our life's beatitude;
Our vain regret are tempered by an inward glow
Whose secret is this same enduring love
From which again springs hope, and hope engenders faith
That this is a beginning - not the end
Of pathways out beyond the stars
This love that kindles hope dispels the bitterness
And soothes the pain of earlier years
Now happy tears may flow again
Our journey's just begun
We little know of life's reality. We have but started to explore
Yet now though dimly through the mists of unbelief
We see a shining goal of unimagined charm
A harbinger, perchance, of immortality.
This fleeting glimpse the passing hour reveals
Is but one word upon a parchment scroll.

A brief eclipse? Maybe, maybe
But after that we shall be free
To seek the greatest of the three great pillars of eternity
A chastened more forbearing love
With sorrows truly shared.

And so, though tears may sometimes flow
They shall not burn.

In reading this one wonders whether "through the mists of unbelief" he felt some guilt at discarding his parents' faith and dedication to God's word, and felt ready to seek the "pillars of eternity." He knew full well that he had made his mark in this world, and maybe, therefore, there was a chance of "immortality" in either this or the next world. Yet despite his success he realised that life fell far short of "unimagined charm." Great sorrow about Hilda Gertrude and James whom he never saw again, must have attended his thoughts, although, as he writes perhaps in denial, not allowed to burn.

Dentistry and the problems of the NHS were never far from his mind and in response to the government White Paper on dentistry in July 1970, he wrote, "I still think, and so do many people that a restricted health service would have many advantages - restricted either as to essential, or as to those that really need it, including, of course, children."

His relationship with Cohen, whom he admired immensely, grew even closer. "What a grand job of it you have made in the Dept." he wrote in a letter in November of that year, and expressed his belief that the Department of Dental Science was an example to other departments of the College, and that they were lucky to have found him (Cohen), and as he wrote in the following January about his own contribution, "...all I ever contributed was to spot the original winner - some fifteen years ago. Well, as Einstein probably thought, we may choose one road but we can't alter what we meet on it."

Einstein was certainly on his mind in the last few years of his life. He knew that his time was drawing in and the nature of that concept occupied his thoughts, thoughts which inevitably, he had to try to sort out and write down.

In the Gospel of St. John, line18.38, Pilate asks of Jesus, "What is truth?", words that must have been very familiar to Fish, and ones that would readily come to mind when answering Colin Davis's question about what he would do if he had his time over again. One can imagine the Reverend Fish using the question about truth as the theme of many a sermon, and when as an elderly man he was interviewed, it seems natural that Fish should be tempted to ring the changes in such a way; truth and time, never ending subjects of philosophic speculation over a dry sherry. Questions about time, and time and relativity theory, came to be the intellectual focus of Fish's interest over these latter years.

Fish had been born into a Newtonian universe where space was a three-dimensional continuum, in which the relationships of locations could be defined by Euclidean postulates, a subject which had been clearly and forcibly enunciated in mathematics classes at Kingswood College. Space had no connection with Time; that was a one-dimensional continuum where 'now' was a point from which duration could be measured into the past and the future. The idea that time is an unfolding of pre-ordained events had been popularised by the philosopher, J.W.Dunne in his book, 'An Experiment with Time' which appeared in 1927, where it was suggested that in dreams we could actually see into the future. Time could be regarded as a continuum of discrete 'nows' or as Fish came to call them 'rolling nows'.

In 1905, during Fish's first year at Kingswood, Einstein published his paper on the Special Theory of Relativity, understood by very few and a source of bewilderment to most. Neither Jules Verne nor H.G.Wells had prepared their readers for such a conceptual earthquake, which redefined physics as the study of the relationship between the observer and events. The idea that two events which appear to occur simultaneously to one observer will be so viewed by all observers irrespective of their location and movement had been disproved. What was observed and what happened was shown to be a function of the observer's location and motion relative to other events. Space and time were one, space-time. Plato's notion of universality was out, relativity was in. Then quantum mechanics introduced further confusion into the mind of the layman.

During Fish's lifetime that earthquake had continued to roll on, and as an intelligent observer of events, in retirement Fish was determined to put his mind to understanding the implications of the new physics. It made a real contrast to concern with the epithelial attachment.

The intriguing subject of time had been discussed with friends in a light-hearted way, giving everyone a chance to produce their own favourite quotations, such as time as a stream that flows over us and ultimately "bears its sons away" and the alternative notion of "we who move through time." No doubt guests left Fish's house with that warm glow which follows such philosophical discussions, but that was not adequate for Fish. He set out to analyse the subject more deeply, and after much reading and contemplation, produced a short book or extended essay which he entitled, 'Just about Time and Relativity'. This represented a great leap from matters of health and oral pathology, and he came to it only as an intelligent layman.

He introduced his own difficulty with the subject, a difficulty shared by most people, by quoting St. Augustine who said," What then is time? If no one asks me I know (but) if I wish to explain it to one that asketh I know not." To that explanation Fish sought help from the dictionary definitions, but finding these inadequate decided that he must try to think the question out for himself and set off on his own voyage of discovery.

He began his thinking and argument with a section that he headed, 'Conjectural Time; a Soliloquy', in which he asked a succession of questions; "did time change everything or did things change anyhow? Did the past still exist - somewhere - or had time swept everything away." "Does tomorrow's sun exist today." Then he asks an even more fundamental question, was there such a thing as time or had we just invented the idea to measure the duration of events and put them in some kind of orderly arrangement?

Ideas of permanence and change follow his first question, writing , "clearly not everything we do or care for ceases to exist as each 'Now' slides into the past." He makes the point that "clearly artifacts have some kind of permanence but emotions, ideas, hopes, which seem just as real as material things when they are experienced, disappear." Aristotle regarded time as an attribute of motion and motion as an attribute of material object, but Fish argues that time is more than material things, "the human concept of the sequence of events is an attribute of the conscious state of the observer not of the events themselves…subjective it may be but the stark fact remains that in everyday life … it is precisely this abstraction that rules our lives."

Fortunately Fish avoided speculation on the nature of reality, a subject that might have driven him into even deeper water, but in considering the 'rolling now' he comments that if this " was the sum total of existence our life would be spent on a constantly moving wave ... on a mere knife edge of infinitely short duration, therefore life would be a nightmare." He pursues the idea that although we cannot see the future except as the Apostle said, "through a glass darkly"... "we believe that we can influence the future by the way we employ this instant of time we call the present ... but the future will soon become the past. Will it (presumably what had been) the future then cease to exist?" In this context Fish quotes the philosopher, Thomas Hobbes (1583-1679), an immensely pragmatic man, who seemed to have no problem with time and avoided all category errors by saying, "The present only has a being in nature, things past have a being in the memory only, but things in the future have no being at all."

Then in looking at predestination, noting that Aristotle accepted an 'open future', Fish asks, "is there anything already established there" (that is in the future). Certainly his upbringing would have emphasised some form of life after death, and perhaps that is the clue to this whole enterprise.

Although struggling with these questions about time, Fish appears to have had no difficulty at all with Einstein's theories and the concept of a four-dimensional continuum, a blend of space and time, and after spelling these ideas out in his own words, asks what might be the practical significance for people in their daily lives of Einstein's theories. This is typical of Fish's attitude to all research; what are its practical implications? How will it affect clinical practice?

Manifestly influenced by the notion of relativity, he then returns to time saying, "it is our own subjective now that divides *our* own past from *our* own future and we cannot share the same now with anyone else who is not in the same rigid reference body with us....we must regard time not as a mere invention of the human mind, concerned to rationalise the observed succession of events; but we must recognize it first as a dimension and then as objectively inseparable from space. In this way time is seen to constitute an essential part of physical reality.

He concludes on a contented note, "it is pleasant to think we live IN time."

Although this writing is manifestly that of a layman swimming in deep and foreign waters, it does demonstrate all Fish's familiar forensic skills, nagging away at the detail of unfamiliar concepts, and teasing out their implications.

He was very keen to see his work published and Cohen put him in touch with the publishers, William Heinemann Medical Books Ltd., whose managing director, Owen R. Evans, passed it on to Tom Rosenthal, managing director of the publishers, Martin Sacker and Warburg, whose opinion they valued highly. Rosenthal was a literary man and not a scientist, and as a layman was very impressed with the manuscript, but on 10th. December 1973 he replied to Heinemann's :

"There is no doubt at all that this is a fascinating piece of writing, full of insights and shafts of wisdom, to a lay reader such as myself, are most impressive.

I must, however, alas read all manuscripts with the possibly permanently jaundiced eye of a literary publisher whose primary emphasis is on fiction, belles lettres and poetry and reluctantly therefore I must tell you that however fascinating and distinguished I personally find the book it would not sit well on our list."

The following day Evans sent a copy of Rosenthal's letter to Fish, who seems to have accepted the rejection philosophically. He had another and more pressing problem to deal with; that was mortality. He knew that the prognosis for the cancer was poor, and that he had not long to live; some time in 1974 he remarked that if Harold Wilson got into power again, he would ask whoever was in charge upstairs to take him.

His failing strength was to frustrate what would have been the fulfilment of the duties of his final public office. As recorded in Chapter 15, the British Society of Periodontology had decided to celebrate its Silver Jubilee meeting of 1974, and to invite Fish to be President for a second time. In tribute to his early research work in periodontology the main theme of the meeting was to be 'The Clinical Application of Microscopic Studies in Periodontology' As always Fish went to a great deal of trouble preparing his presidential address, starting his preparation in the previous year. He wrote to Cohen to obtain slides from the Department of Dental Science, and in order to bring his facts up-to-date he obtained the latest book on the subject, 'Fine Structure of the Epithelial Attachment' by Schroeder and Listgarten, at that time two of the most eminent workers in the field. The foreword to the book had been written by Frank G. Everett, a former student of Gottlieb, to whom Fish owed a great deal in his early research on periodontal disease. By this route Fish was completing a circle.

Although at this time he claimed to be feeling quite well, and in April 1973 he had even bought a large new car, an Austin Maxi, to accommodate himself, Hazel and their three dogs, his condition was deteriorating. Early in 1974 his daughter Vivien, his favourite child, came from New Zealand to see him for the last time.

Despite his failing health he pursued his regular correspondence with Cohen as well as attending the occasional social function, and in one 'thank you' letter to Cohen, expressed his gratitude for Cohen's suggestion that there be a Fish laboratory at Downe. Inevitably he continued to nag at the precise cause of periodontal disease, and still doubtful of the role of bacterial plaque, in March 1974, he put to Cohen a question about any contact of subgingival plaque with the junction of the oral and junctional epithelia, and continued, "I would have thought not - but 'Don't think', I can hear you say, 'Try the experiment', - well I will if they have teeth to grind in Hell !."

In the same month Fish wrote to Cohen, "You must on no account let your report on pyorrhoea research ....slip onto the dusty shelves."

Also he was not yet finished with a subject that he had always preached about, that is the relationship between research and clinical practice. As Bowen has pointed out, he was heavily committed to what is now known as 'transitional research', that is research that could be readily applied to the clinical situation, and he was concerned about the public rift that had appeared between dentists in practice and research workers. An editorial regretting this situation had appeared in the BDJ of April 16th.1974, which provoked Fish to reply, "May I be permitted to congratulate you very sincerely on your editorial...deploring the 'mild but definite antipathy' and the 'lack of understanding' between clinicians and research workers. This sad state of affairs must at all costs be remedied."

The officers of the BSP were in continual contact with him, but their plans were not to be fulfilled. The Silver Jubilee meeting was held at the Royal College of Surgeons without their President. Fish died at his home in Storrington on July 20th. 1974 and the funeral was held at Worthing crematorium. A memorial service attended by many old students, colleagues and friends was held on Wednesday, November 12th. at St. Marylebone Parish Church on the Marylebone Road, behind which Charles Wesley is buried. The service was conducted by the Reverend Dr. F. Coventry and the Reading was given by David Hindley-Smith, Registrar of the General Dental Council.

Sir Robert Bradlaw, then President of the British Dental Association, gave a short address in which he said that the occasion was not one for a panegyric but to remember and pay tribute to a man and to a friend who had rendered such great service to his profession.

Chapter 18

THE MAJOR PLAYER

Professor H.M.Pickard, a student, then colleague and friend of Fish, and therefore someone who had known him for many years and in many roles, wrote about his teacher, "In a profession, which does not, I believe, attract men of the highest intellect, Fish was an intellectual well above the majority of his colleagues and in my experience, the most intellectually demanding and stimulating of any of the leaders of the dental profession with whom I have come into contact. I felt, I readily admit, that his mind leapt from mountain peak to mountain peak, whilst I was left laboriously scrambling down one side and up the other, of the valleys of understanding which he crossed so effortlessly." Pickard, who was among the first group of full-time teachers at the Royal Dental Hospital, believed that Fish was never really at ease there despite the fact that the twelve years he spent at the RDH, in teaching and research, were amongst the most productive of Fish's career. In his work on denture design, the physiology of the dental tissues, and more particularly in his conclusions about focal infection, he must have crossed swords all too often with the old-guard on the medical and management committees, but it was in the matter of research funding that differences were most obvious. Fish did not suffer fools gladly, and the manner of his departure from the RDH is testimony to both ill-feeling and to the reluctance of many of his peers, who were, after all, leaders of the profession, to change their ideas and modify their practices.

It is difficult to accept the transience of ideas. In any work, the daily routine revolves around a focus of accepted beliefs which provides foundation and anchor for practice, but also shackle. A clear example of this is the resistance put up by surgeons to Lister's antiseptic techniques on the basis that his life saving methods obscured much of the skill of surgery, this despite the overwhelming evidence of Lister's success. It is also too easy to take our current body of knowledge for granted, and even to assume that what we know is the result of a seamless unravelling of fact and understanding that took place without error and confusion, let alone disappointment. Today's dentistry, like all bodies of knowledge and practice, was built brick by brick, some sliding easily into place while others required considerable demolition of firmly held ideas and procedures before they sat comfortably.

As he had shown in childhood, one of Fish's strongest character traits was curiosity. Questioning why things should be so was evident when as a student of both medicine and dentistry, he asked himself why we could put infected filling material into living, that is sensitive, dentine, whereas the slightest infection introduced as a foreign body into bone caused an abscess. In answering such questions he found many walls to knock down, not least the ignorance of his teachers, one of whom could only reply that he should get on with his work and not ask so many questions. His thinking was characterised by his ability to ask simple and basic questions, e.g. where is the evidence of fluid flow through enamel if it is a vital tissue? And to that end he applied rigorous research methods, as exemplified by his clarification of the pathology of the apical root lesion, and once he was convinced of the correctness of his theses, he pronounced them repeatedly and at length, with clarity, eloquence and conviction.

Despite his upbringing Fish had little interest in religion. Nevertheless he brought to his work and his efforts on behalf of his profession the zeal of a crusader. He was on a mission. The earliest lessons of the only son of a Wesleyan minister and his evangelical wife were those of faith, duty and hard work: faith in a God who was not always benevolent, but in whom one must put one's trust; belief in one's duty to serve Him, and to serve the community by spreading His Word, which was the Gospel; and the conviction that the way to achieve one's objectives was by a regular systematic way of thinking and behaving. Every day was ordered to a purpose.

Despite the changes in social and personal values of the early part of the twentieth century, in which the Great War played such a crucial part, this devotion to systematic thought, diligence and decorum as lived by his parents, remained at the root of Fish's life and work.

His parents' dedication and hard work were models for his own, his father's preaching an example for his own teaching. By his son's account, the Reverend Fish was not a practical man. He left the repair of his bicycle tyres to the young Fish. Nor could the minister bear the sight of blood, and his son's experiments on tiddlers could not be carried out in his presence. So Eric Wilfred, with two sisters and an indulgent mother, became the useful male in the household, and no doubt received due admiration and acknowledgement for his curiosity and achievements. He certainly had confidence in his own ability, a confidence fortified by successful performances at school and in his professional education. His readiness to articulate his views and to challenge the views of his colleagues whatever their seniority, led to charges of arrogance.

Deference was not something he found easy; nor did he expect it. Honesty was a central virtue of his parents' lives and drilled into Fish by example and teaching. A story demonstrating his honesty and integrity was provided by E.R.Briault in an appreciation after Fish's death. Briault had sent a patient to Fish for an opinion, and Fish made a diagnosis and wrote out an opinion. This was typed, but before posting the letter Fish changed his mind and wrote a different recommendation. However he sent both opinions to Briault to show that even he could get it wrong. A further example, so the story goes, arose just before he retired. His colleagues at the practice in Cavendish Square decided that the premises needed refurbishing, and to that end patients might be asked to pay in cash. Fish was adamant that this was wrong , and that all earnings must be declared in full. Kingswood School was the right school for a bright boy. Kingswood boys had a reputation for doing brilliantly at university, in particular at London University at a time when Nonconformists were not accepted at Oxford and Cambridge. Thomas Arnold, the great headmaster of Rugby School, set three markers for his boys, religious and moral principles, gentlemanly conduct, and intellectual ability, and thus set the tone for the Victorian Public Schools, including Kingswood. John Wesley taught as part of the Methodist creed, the equality of all under God, and concern for the under privileged. During Fish's time as a pupil at Kingswood, the then Governor, W.P. Workman, preached, "Life as a whole is given to save others and to help others, you cannot possibly spare yourself." While never a Socialist, indeed there is no evidence that he ever took any real interest in politics, Fish seems to have been a natural egalitarian at a time when manifestations of class differences defined behaviour to other people. He met his cleaner or any other of his employees, on equal terms; the quality of their work was what mattered, and whenever that was at issue he spoke frankly.

From an early age Fish wanted to be a doctor. Accompanying his father on his pastoral duties opened his eyes to the ever-present manifestations of poverty and disease, and it might have been a disappointment to him to be enrolled as a student in what was perceived then as an inferior profession to medicine. A great many of his fellow students had been apprenticed as dental mechanics, as had many of his teachers at the start of their careers, and he must have felt that here he was, a prizeman from a scholarly institution, and well versed in the classics, aligned with less well educated, and no doubt less intelligent young men. However he never expressed any disappointment at his start in dentistry, and his teachers seem to have recognised that he was a special student. It will have been no surprise to anyone that despite by-passing the official channels for registering for the medical course, along with his friend, H.H.Stones, he had no difficulty in that regard. It is interesting that because Stones was on the BDS course, he qualified a year ahead of Fish, who had been on the LDS course.

Also the intensely practical nature of the dental training accorded with Fish's own natural aptitude for solving technical problems, and whatever he felt about the intellectual demands of the dental course, meeting the many challenges of the mechanics laboratory must have provided great satisfaction. His drawing and photographic skills, and later his histological work, are testimony to these talents. Bert Cohen, Fish's colleague at the Department of Dental Science, has described how when Fish visited the Cohens' new but not yet furnished house, Fish made a ceiling rose for a light fitting. There and then he commanded paper and water, made papier-mache, and moulded it into a ceiling rose which adorned the Cohen's ceiling for years. Leaving the love and warmth of the family home to go to boarding school at the age of ten must have been a great wrench and the cause of the loneliness that his wife, Hazel, says he felt at school. but it did not seem to affect his ability to make friends later in life. Despite the reserve in his character, a feature that several people including his former students, Pickard and Miles have commented on, perhaps enhanced by an appearance of aloofness given by his high-domed Nordic features, he made many friends, if not intimates, throughout his life, and because of his own self-confidence and belief in his work, he inspired enthusiasm, confidence and friendship in those who worked with him. Many of the connections that Fish made early in his career became important to him later in life. One of these was H.A. Harris, who had taught physics before going into medicine, and was to become Professor of Anatomy at Cambridge. He was Senior Demonstrator in the anatomy department at UCL when Fish carried out the research for his MD, and had a special link with Fish. Harris had been the son of a struggling widow in Merthyr Tydfil in Wales, where he had gone to elementary and secondary school, and therefore like Fish had a Noncomformist background. Just as Pickard thought that Fish was never at ease at the RDH, so Cohen felt that there were occasions at the Royal College of Surgeons when Fish did not seem completely at home. When he presided at dinners of the Board of the Faculty of Dental Surgery he was in his element, but during academic committee meetings or in discussion with non-dental academic colleagues he was less at ease. Perhaps in those contexts he felt less of a true scientist, but those were days of class consciousness, and maybe as the graduate of a red-brick university he was not at ease with the products of Oxford and Cambridge. However another social explanation seems possible. At the beginning of the twentieth century a Nonconformist clergyman would have been ranked in the lower middle class with perhaps a finger touch on the margins of the middle class. Certainly they were not among the affluent members of the professions, and Fish's intimacy with H.A.Harris, a man of a similar background may provide a clue to a residuum of class feeling. But at a deeper level Fish was not a team player, unless of course he led the team, as his father had led his Wesleyan flock. In reading Fish's addresses to the Dental Board and then to the General Dental Council it is easy to hear the cleric delivering the regular Sabbath sermon. Cohen has commented that Fish liked to lay down the rules and found it difficult to conform to rules laid down by others, and perhaps in this Fish was extending the boundaries of the Nonconformist attitude. Certainly in his research he was reluctant to accept a theory or traditional practice as a given before he had tested it to his satisfaction.

Another early contact was (later Sir) Charles Lovatt Evans, who became the Professor of Physiology at UCL at the time Fish was carrying out the research on the physiology of the dental tissues. Almost twenty years later as Chairman of the Dental Selection Committee, Evans played an important role in the Faculty of Dental Surgery and the Department of Dental Science. Fleming and MacLean, Fish's colleagues at St. Mary's, also became friends.

It was common then, as it still is, for professional people to make good use of the influence of their clients or patients, and with a celebrity practice Fish became an expert at that art.

Beaverbrook, Churchill and Brendan Bracken were among those who played an important role in Fish's life, and while at St. Mary's, Fish recruited the support of his patient, the Jewish philanthropist, Edward Meyerstein, to found the Dental Research Laboratory there.

Fish also had a gift for recognising an opportunity when he met one, and he recognised opportunities in Sevenoaks and in UCL, the two important springboards for his career. The potential of Sevenoaks as a pleasant place to live and establish a successful practice may well have been prompted by Colyer, Fish's hospital chief at that time, but Fish did not hesitate and by 1920 was well esconced. There for almost twenty years he built the backbone of his financial security, a practice which as Eustace and Partners still prospers. At the same time as he set up in practice he discovered that one did not need to be on the official staff of UCL to carry out research there. One could pay for the use of the laboratory facilities there, so Fish became an honorary researcher to work for his MD.

H.H. Stones was a lifelong friend, and a comparison between the two men helps to underline some of the characteristics of Fish's personality. Photographs of the two men together at meetings show Stones rather undistinguished in appearance, informally dressed and relaxed, while Fish appears very formal, rather cold, and alert to his surroundings. Despite qualifying in medicine before Fish, Stones obtained his MD four years after Fish, and the research that Stones carried out for his MD was at the Hampton Hale Laboratory on periodontal pathology where Fish already directed the department.

Stones was a friendly, quiet and scholarly man, essentially a research worker who, despite becoming Director of the Liverpool Dental School, disliked administration. He admired Fish, who was a dynamic administrator and organiser to the point of obsession. Fish's preparatory notes for lectures and papers are detailed and meticulous. Where facts were needed he had all those and the figures to confirm them, and his main themes were repeated again and again. This was especially the case when it came to his primary concern on the Dental Board, the training of teachers and research workers. The avuncular side to Fish's nature comes out in his relationships with his juniors, and in particular in his relations with Stewart Ross, probably his closest friend. Ross his senior assistant and then partner in the practices in Sevenoaks and Cavendish Square, was also Fish's assistant at the Hampton Hale Laboratory. MacRoss, as everyone called him, was, as Gerald Leatherman was to write in his obituary, a kind and patient man, not ambitious, and never wanting to take centre stage, in short a perfect companion for his mentor, whom he also followed in his political activity at the FDI and the GDC. They went deer stalking together, and despite being only a decade younger, in many ways Ross seems to have been a surrogate son to replace James, the son who had been such a disappointment to Fish. But Fish was not the father that James could emulate. Dedication to his professional activity absorbed Fish's life, even when he was at home. It destroyed his first marriage and the woman who had joined herself to him when both were too young, and then alienated his son for whom rebellion was the only course. By the time of his second marriage in 1950 Fish had achieved considerable national and international success, to be crowned two years later by his presidency of the XIth. International Dental Congress in London. Hazel was an attractive and vivacious widow, almost twenty years Fish's junior, and with her background in the world of art she brought a new dimension into Fish's life that he was to enjoy to the end. They had known each other for many years, and indeed Hazel's first husband, the painter Francis Hodge, actually taught Fish to paint, and Hazel claimed that Fish could have been a very good painter if he had put his mind to it.

Fish's attitude to women is revealed in a letter that he wrote to The Times in 1964, in which he states, "Cannot we provide in the welfare state, which seems somehow to have upset family tradition of preparing children for life's responsibilities, to keep young women at home and train them, if they already do not know how, to inculcate unselfish and respectful habits of conduct in their children? It would be a better investment than offering higher education to young people with no sense of moral obligations."

Although he was then seventy his views almost certainly reflect the views of most men of all ages at that time. As a young man in 1936 Fish had been the one to represent the view of the Medical Committee when he moved the resolution to ban the further intake of women to the RDH.

Hazel Fish has described how keen he was for her to dress on special occasions according to his wishes, and it seems likely that he dominated his less independent first wife even more strictly. That he felt the need to be sure that his wives adequately reflected his status again suggests some insecurity about his place in society. However he was always at ease with his dental colleagues.

Fish's two marriages were symbolic of two phases of his life, the ascent of the ladder and his arrival at the top, and these phases coincided roughly with the two periods in the development of his profession, the pre- and post-war periods.

In the pre-war period, from the 1921 Dental Act, the evolution of the profession was slow, and throughout that time it was formally within the orbit of the General Medical Council. Even though the Dental Board had responsibility for funding dental education and research, the GMC had a say in the structure of the dental curriculum and the inspection of dental schools. It was a time when the responsibility of government, and therefore of the Ministry of Health was limited. The Department of Education and Local Education Authorities had responsibility for the school dental clinics, but in every other respect, registration, discipline, training and research, the burden fell, via the Dental Board, onto the profession. In fact the profession supported itself. Any additional financial support was provided by the generosity of benefactors. In this way Fish's own research was funded when the money didn't actually come out of his own pocket. The largest benefactor to dentistry, Lord Nuffield, was not yet on the scene. Before 1939 Fish's reputation derived from his scientific activity which he reported regularly in the journals, mainly the BDJ and the Proceedings of the Royal Society of Medicine. No other scientific worker in dentistry at that time received the exposure that Fish commanded.

His lectures and articles about his research were accessible to all. He engendered enormous enthusiasm for the work in his co-workers and students, and often said that enthusiasm was essential to the research worker. Appropriately he quoted Pasteur who said, " The Greeks have given us one of the most beautiful words known to Man. Enthusiasm, a god within. Blessed is he who possesses a god within." Enthusiasm was one of his strongest traits.

In describing his work he progressed in clear and logical sequences from an account of basic physiology and pathology through the steps of his investigation to a conclusion that by then seemed to his audience as inevitable. He represented, as did no-one else of his time, the progress of dental science. Through years of painstaking research he had demolished the Mellanby theory of the causation of dental caries, lent a new dimension to denture design, and shed light on the influence of dental pathology on dental health. It came as no surprise that his election in 1939 to the Dental Board came with an overwhelming majority. In making Fish an honorary member of their dental associations Australia and the Netherlands had already recognised his worth. It was not long before the Privy Council also recognised his political ability by appointing him Chairman of the Dental Board to steer the profession through to increasing independence from medicine. After the war there were other important and influential figures on the scene, such as Kelsey Fry and Wilkinson, but only Bradlaw could be said to rank with Fish as a star in the dental firmament.

Kelsey Fry, through his connections with general and plastic surgeons from the First World War, was instrumental in establishing that branch of dental surgeons who became known as oral and maxillo-facial surgeons. According to Miles he was unimpressive in manner and speech, but very effective behind the scenes. He was an excellent committee member who had a reputation for getting his own way, especially on a one-to-one basis, and as a government advisor he was very influential. Wilkinson was a powerful administrator, who as the Dean of three dental schools, Melbourne, Manchester and then the Eastman, made these comparatively new institutions into effective teaching and treatment machines. Two of his former House Surgeons, A.W.Moule and T.F.Monks said that when Wilkinson arrived at Manchester Dental Hospital in 1933, the staff felt as though a typhoon had hit them. Dynamic and at times ruthless, he had the capacity to build loyal teams. As described in his obituary, he had those qualities that make captains, but neither he nor Kelsey Fry seem to have possessed the wider imagination to make good generals.

In the nineteen thirties the Honoraries held a firm grip on undergraduate teaching, especially in the London schools, and at Newcastle Bradlaw placed teaching in the committed hands of the full-time teachers. He was not the only one to make such changes. At Birmingham, Professor Humphrey Humphreys, who in 1935 became the first professor of dental surgery, then Dean of the Dental School and subsequently Vice-Chancellor of the University, had by 1949 three full-time professors on his staff. In this important move the provincial schools led the way, but Humphreys was never tempted away from Birmingham and the Midlands. Bradlaw brought his powerful personality and wit to the field of dental education, and to the initiation of the Fellowship in Dental Surgery of the Royal College of Surgeons of England. He saw, as did Fish, that if dentistry was to achieve anything like parity of status with other branches of medicine it must be made up of rigorously trained professional people. But like Kelsey Fry and Wilkinson he made little contribution to dental science. The panorama of Fish's activity was much wider than that of any of his contemporaries, and his years, twenty-five in all, at the Dental Board and then the General Dental Council, saw the emergence of a dental statesman. His emphasis on training teachers and research workers was not simply to provide Britain with a better dental service. The centre of Fish's programme was like Bradlaw's, to improve the status of dentistry as a respected profession that could stand on equal terms by the side of other medical and surgical specialities.

Only by basing dental practice on sound scientific foundations could this be achieved, and perhaps Fish's greatest claim to fame rests on the fact that in both the clinical and research domains his work altered everyday dental practice in prosthetics, periodontal treatment, as well as in the dramatic change in attitude within both dentistry and medicine to oral sepsis. None of his peers could claim eponymous instruments or techniques, or to have exerted such influence on both the dental profession and the general public in the practice of oral hygiene. In his own person at the RCS he was seen as an equal amongst the best in surgery. No one in dentistry since John Tomes exerted such a wide influence, or held the reins of power for so long. The parallel between the two men has been well recognised in both medicine and dentistry, a comparability that was perfectly if crudely expressed in the following piece of comic verse recited by the eminent surgeon, Sir Vincent Zachary Cope, in 1959 at a dinner of the Board of the Faculty of Dental Surgery at the Royal College of Surgeons. Sir Z, as he was known, was the author of a biography of John Tomes, and of a popular book, 'Florence Nightingale and the Doctors'.

His verse went:

> " To fight disease we need
> increase of knowledge,
> Fruitful research is what we
> All now wish.
> In this great faculty within
> The College
> Research is thriving, thanks
> To Wilfred Fish.
> If you would seek the birth of
> Your profession
> You do not need the help of
> Sherlock Holmes
> For it is agreed by general
> Concession
> The midwife at the birth
> Was Johnnie Tomes. "

John Tomes died on the 29th. July 1895, eighteen months after Fish was born, and in the continuity of the lives of these two men can be traced the making of a profession. Many others played important roles , men of foresight, drive and administrative skills, but Tomes and Fish were visionaries and crusaders in their aspirations for their profession. Tomes pressed for a Royal Charter to introduce a department of dental surgery at the

RCS, and to establish examinations for a legal qualification to practise dentistry, and finally in the face of opposition from medicine, to bring about the Dental Act of 1878, and Fish managed the Dental Board to its natural fulfilment in the General Dental Council. They inspired their peers and successors to an aspiration which in large part has been fulfilled. Within the family of the Royal College of Surgeons of England they were the true heirs of John Hunter. With the growth of specialisation it is most unlikely that we shall see their like again.